New Medical Technology in Patient Care

A Physician's Guide

Other Titles by the Author

Fascinating Fringes of Medicine: From Oddities to Innovations
ISBN: 978-981-12-8407-6
ISBN: 978-981-12-8455-7 (pbk)

Artificial Intelligence in Medicine: A Practical Guide for Clinicians
ISBN: 978-981-12-8410-6
ISBN: 978-981-12-8456-4 (pbk)

In the Name of Progress: The Dark Side of Medical Research
ISBN: 978-981-12-9181-4

New Medical Technology in Patient Care

A Physician's Guide

Campion Quinn, MD

Rockville Medical, LLC, USA

World Scientific

NEW JERSEY · LONDON · SINGAPORE · BEIJING · SHANGHAI · TAIPEI · CHENNAI

Published by

World Scientific Publishing Co. Pte. Ltd.

5 Toh Tuck Link, Singapore 596224

USA office: 27 Warren Street, Suite 401-402, Hackensack, NJ 07601

UK office: 57 Shelton Street, Covent Garden, London WC2H 9HE

Library of Congress Control Number: 2024060696

British Library Cataloguing-in-Publication Data
A catalogue record for this book is available from the British Library.

NEW MEDICAL TECHNOLOGY IN PATIENT CARE
A Physician's Guide

ISBN 978-981-12-8914-9 (hardcover)
ISBN 978-981-12-8915-6 (ebook for institutions)
ISBN 978-981-12-8916-3 (ebook for individuals)

For any available supplementary material, please visit
https://www.worldscientific.com/worldscibooks/10.1142/13753#t=suppl

Desk Editor: Brittney Phitojo

Typeset by Stallion Press
Email: enquiries@stallionpress.com

To my wife, Nancy, for everything

Contents

Introduction

New Medical Technology in Patient Care: A Physician's Guide embarks on an enlightening journey through medical technology's dynamic and rapidly evolving world. This book is a meticulously crafted mosaic of the latest advancements, innovations, and breakthroughs in healthcare and medical research. It serves as a comprehensive guide and an insightful exploration into how these technological marvels are not just revolutionizing patient care and treatment methodologies, but also challenging and redefining the traditional paradigms of medical research and practice.

The chapters of this book are thoughtfully curated to provide readers with a panoramic view of contemporary medical technologies. Each chapter delves into a specific area of medical technology, offering in-depth insights into its current state, potential applications, challenges, and future prospects. From the intricacies of genomics and personalized medicine to the cutting-edge developments in organ-on-a-chip technology, this book covers a broad spectrum of topics at the forefront of medical innovation.

Our journey begins with exploring the transformative world of genomics and personalized medicine. Here, we delve into how the customization of healthcare, based on individual genetic profiles, is becoming a tangible reality, promising treatments and therapies that are precisely tailored to each patient's unique genetic makeup. This chapter not only explores the scientific and technological aspects of genomics but also addresses these advancements' ethical, legal, and societal implications.

We then navigate through the groundbreaking realm of organ-on-a-chip technology. This marvel of bioengineering, which integrates microfabrication with tissue engineering, promises to revolutionize drug development, disease modeling, and our understanding of human physiology. The chapter dedicated to this topic elucidates how these microfluidic devices, which emulate human organ functions, are set to transform pharmaceutical research and offer more accurate models for disease studies.

As the book progresses, readers are introduced to the innovative world of wearable health monitors and mobile health applications. These chapters highlight how technology increasingly intertwines with our daily lives, offering new health monitoring, disease prevention, and management avenues. The discussion extends to the impact of these technologies on patient engagement, healthcare delivery, and the potential for a more proactive approach to health and wellness.

Another significant focus of this book is integrating artificial intelligence (AI) in healthcare. This section delves into how AI and machine learning are leveraged to enhance diagnostic accuracy, personalize treatment plans, and improve patient outcomes. It also examines the challenges and ethical considerations associated with the deployment of AI in medical settings.

New Medical Technology in Patient Care is not just a compilation of technological advancements; it is a narrative that weaves together these innovations' potential, challenges, and ethical considerations. It is designed to cater to a diverse audience, including medical professionals, researchers, students, and technology enthusiasts. Each chapter is crafted to be accessible yet informative, ensuring that readers from various backgrounds can appreciate the depth and breadth of medical technology.

This book is an invitation to explore the fascinating world of medical technology. It encourages readers to contemplate the vast possibilities, address the challenges, and acknowledge the responsibilities accompanying these advancements. As we stand on the brink of a new era in healthcare, *New Medical Technology in Patient Care: A Physician's Guide* offers a glimpse into a future where technology and healthcare converge to improve lives and redefine the boundaries of medical science.

Chapter 1

AI for Accurate Diagnosis

AI represents a groundbreaking advancement in healthcare, promising a transformative impact on patient care through precise diagnostic capabilities. This chapter explores the dynamic landscape of AI applications focused on analyzing medical images, electronic health records (EHRs) data, and diagnostic tests. Integrating AI technologies in these domains offers numerous advantages, including early disease detection and reduced diagnostic errors, ultimately enhancing patient outcomes.

AI Applications in Analyzing Medical Images, EHR Data, and Diagnostic Tests

Medical Imaging Analysis

AI technologies have significantly impacted medical imaging. These technologies have paved the way for a more efficient and precise interpretation of various medical images, including X-rays, magnetic resonance imaging (MRIs), computed tomography (CT) scans, and ultrasounds. This section explores the critical AI applications in this domain and their significant advantages.

AI's integration in medical imaging involves the development of sophisticated algorithms capable of interpreting various types of medical images, including X-rays, MRIs, CT scans, and more. These algorithms use deep learning techniques to recognize patterns and anomalies, aiding in the accurate and timely diagnosis of conditions. For instance, AI algorithms can identify subtle signs of potential tumors, fractures, or abnormalities that might be difficult to detect with the human eye alone.

Deep Learning in Medical Imaging

Deep learning algorithms are at the forefront of AI's integration into medical imaging. These algorithms use neural networks to recognize intricate patterns and anomalies in medical images. Their ability to process vast amounts of data allows for the early detection of conditions that might be difficult for human radiologists to identify. For example, AI algorithms can identify subtle signs of potential tumors, fractures, or abnormalities that might be missed by the human eye alone.

Improving Radiology Workflow

AI-driven solutions have the potential to streamline radiology workflows, reducing the time it takes to interpret images and deliver results. This improves efficiency and allows for more timely diagnosis and treatment, which is particularly crucial in emergencies.

AI Applications in EHR Data Analysis

Unlocking the Potential of EHRs

EHRs serve as comprehensive patient data repositories, including medical history, medications, lab results, treatment plans, and more. AI algorithms can unlock the valuable insights hidden within these digital records, aiding healthcare professionals in making informed decisions.

Natural Language Processing in EHR Analysis

Natural language processing (NLP) algorithms are pivotal in extracting structured information from an unstructured text within EHRs. This capability provides a comprehensive overview of a patient's health history, facilitating personalized treatment planning and continuous monitoring. NLP also enhances data accessibility for researchers and policymakers.

AI Applications in Diagnostic Test Analysis

Enhancing Diagnostic Accuracy

AI can significantly enhance the accuracy and efficiency of diagnostic test interpretation. Machine learning (ML) models can process vast datasets generated from various diagnostic tests, including blood tests, genetic screenings, and biomarker analyses. By identifying subtle markers and patterns within these datasets, AI can assist in early disease detection and more precise diagnosis, enabling proactive and targeted treatment approaches.

Predictive Analytics

Beyond diagnosis, AI can also play a crucial role in predictive analytics. AI models can predict disease risk and progression by analyzing a patient's historical data and trends, allowing for preventive interventions and personalized treatment plans.

Conclusion

The integration of AI in healthcare, particularly in medical imaging, EHR data analysis, and diagnostic test interpretation, represents a significant advancement in modern medicine. These applications offer a promising future in early disease detection, reduced diagnostic errors, and improved patient outcomes. As AI continues to evolve, its role in healthcare is poised to expand further, bringing us closer to the vision of precision medicine.

Introduction to Revolutionizing Medicine with AI: The Power of Medical Image Analysis

In modern healthcare, medical imaging is indisputably pivotal. It serves as a window into the human body, enabling healthcare professionals to visualize, diagnose, and monitor various medical conditions. Medical imaging has revolutionized diagnosis, treatment, and patient care, from detecting cancerous tumors to evaluating the integrity of bones and organs. However, the sheer complexity and volume of medical image data have presented formidable challenges for traditional methods of analysis and interpretation.

As we embark on this journey into the profound transformation brought about by AI, we find ourselves at the intersection of cutting-edge technology and the practice of medicine. The AI revolution, particularly in the context of medical image analysis, represents a monumental leap forward in our ability to harness the potential of these visual insights for the betterment of healthcare.

Setting the Stage: The Role of Medical Imaging in Modern Healthcare

The significance of medical imaging in modern healthcare cannot be overstated. It has become integral to clinical decision-making, research, and patient care across various medical disciplines. Here, we delve into the multifaceted role that medical imaging plays:

1. Diagnosis and Disease Detection

Medical imaging techniques such as X-rays, CT scans, and MRI have become indispensable tools for diagnosing various medical conditions. Whether it's identifying a fractured bone, detecting the early stages of cancer, or evaluating the progression of neurological disorders, medical images provide crucial information that forms the foundation of clinical decision-making.

2. Treatment Planning and Monitoring

Beyond diagnosis, medical imaging guides treatment strategies. Surgeons rely on precise imaging to plan and execute procedures with minimal invasiveness. Radiation therapy and chemotherapy regimens are tailored based on imaging data. Additionally, medical images facilitate real-time monitoring of treatment response, enabling adjustments as needed.

3. Research and Advancements

Medical imaging fuels research and innovation. It allows scientists to study disease mechanisms, track the efficacy of new therapies, and explore the intricacies of the human body. Advances in imaging technology often pave the way for breakthroughs in medical science.

4. Patient-Centered Care

From a patient's perspective, medical imaging provides clarity and insight into their health. It helps demystify medical conditions and empowers individuals to participate actively in healthcare decisions. In essence, medical images bridge the gap between the abstract and the tangible, making health concerns more comprehensible.

The AI Revolution: How AI is Transforming Medical Image Analysis

As we stand on the brink of the AI revolution, it's essential to grasp the profound impact this technology has on medical image analysis. AI, driven by sophisticated algorithms and ML models, possesses the potential to revolutionize the way we interpret and derive insights from medical images.

1. Precision and Efficiency

AI algorithms can analyze vast datasets of medical images with unparalleled precision and speed. They excel at recognizing subtle patterns, anomalies, and abnormalities that might elude even the most experienced human radiologists. This heightened precision enhances diagnostic accuracy and expedites the entire process, allowing for more timely intervention when needed.

2. Personalized Medicine

AI can tailor medical treatment plans to individual patients, recommend personalized therapies, and predict treatment outcomes by analyzing medical images in conjunction with patient-specific data. This approach marks a shift from one-size-fits-all medicine to patient-centered, precision medicine.

3. Augmenting Healthcare Professionals

Rather than replacing healthcare professionals, AI complements their expertise. It is a powerful tool for radiologists, clinicians, and surgeons, providing valuable insights and assisting in decision-making. This collaborative approach ensures that the human touch remains at the core of healthcare.

The Scope of this Chapter: A Preview of AI Applications in Medical Image Analysis

In the following chapters, we will delve deeper into the fascinating world of AI applications in medical image analysis. From the fundamentals of deep learning and convolutional neural networks (CNNs) to real-world case studies showcasing AI's impact on diagnosis and treatment, we will explore the multifaceted landscape of AI-powered medical imaging. Moreover, we will examine the challenges and ethical considerations accompanying this technological revolution and ponder the future directions and innovations.

Join us as we embark on this journey through medical imaging and AI convergence. This journey promises to improve patient care, advance medical science, and redefine the boundaries of what is possible in modern healthcare.

Fundamentals of Medical Imaging

An Overview of Medical Imaging Modalities

Before delving into the transformative role of AI in medical image analysis, it is essential to understand the diverse range of medical imaging modalities that serve as the foundation for diagnosis and treatment in modern healthcare.

X-rays

X-rays are a fundamental imaging technique that uses ionizing radiation to create images of the body's internal structures. They are commonly employed to visualize bones, detect fractures, and assess the condition of the chest and lungs. X-ray images, or radiographs, are grayscale representations, with denser tissues appearing brighter.

Magnetic Resonance Imaging

MRI, based on the principles of magnetic resonance, produces highly detailed images of soft tissues, including the brain, muscles, and internal organs. Unlike X-rays, MRI does not use ionizing radiation but relies on strong magnetic fields and radio waves. MRI provides exquisite contrast resolution and is particularly useful for visualizing neurological and musculoskeletal structures.

CT Scans

CT scans combine X-ray technology with computer processing to generate cross-sectional images of the body. These images, called slices or tomograms, allow for a detailed examination of internal structures from various angles. CT scans are vital in diagnosing conditions such as tumors, vascular diseases, and injuries.

Ultrasound

Ultrasound imaging, or sonography, employs high-frequency sound waves to produce real-time images of organs, blood vessels, and developing fetuses. It is noninvasive and widely used in obstetrics, cardiology and in assessing abdominal and pelvic structures. Ultrasound offers real-time visualization and is an essential tool in prenatal care.

Nuclear Medicine Imaging

Nuclear medicine imaging involves introducing radioactive materials, known as radiopharmaceuticals, into the body. Specialized cameras capture the emissions of gamma rays from these radioactive tracers, creating images that reflect physiological processes. This modality is used for diagnosing and monitoring conditions such as cancer, heart disease, and thyroid disorders.

Importance of Image Quality and Resolution

The quality and resolution of medical images play a critical role in accurate diagnosis and treatment planning. High-resolution images provide fine details, enabling healthcare professionals to identify subtle abnormalities and make precise measurements. Image quality is influenced by factors such as the imaging technique, equipment specifications, and patient preparation.

Challenges in Traditional Image Interpretation

Traditional image interpretation relies on the expertise of radiologists and clinicians. However, highly skilled human interpreters face the following challenges:

- Subjectivity: Interpretation can be subjective, varying from one expert to another.
- Fatigue: Prolonged viewing of images may lead to fatigue, affecting accuracy.
- Workload: The increasing volume of medical images poses challenges in timely interpretation.
- Complexity: Certain conditions require extensive detection experience; even experts may miss subtle findings.

The integration of AI in medical image analysis addresses these challenges by offering objectivity, consistency, and efficiency. In the following sections, we will explore how AI and profound learning algorithms enhance the capabilities of medical imaging across these modalities and addresses these longstanding challenges.

Understanding AI in Healthcare

Before we explore AI's role in medical image analysis, we must grasp the fundamentals of AI in healthcare.

AI, a branch of computer science, focuses on creating intelligent systems capable of performing tasks that typically require human intelligence. In healthcare, AI encompasses a range of techniques, including ML, deep learning, NLP, and computer vision. These techniques enable AI systems to analyze large datasets, derive meaningful insights, and make informed decisions.

Artificial Intelligence (AI)
↓
Machine Learning (ML)
↙   ↘
Deep Learning   NLP and Computer vision
↓
Convolutional Neural Networks (CNNs)

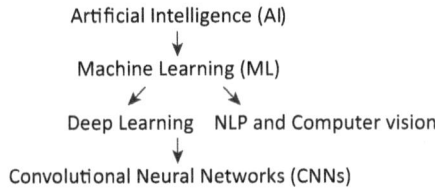

Artificial Intelligence (AI):	AI is the overarching field focused on creating intelligent systems that can perform tasks that typically require human intelligence. It encompasses various subfields, including ML.
Machine Learning (ML):	ML is a subset of AI that concentrates on the development of algorithms and models that allow computers to learn from data and improve their performance on tasks through experience without human programming.
Deep Learning:	Deep learning is a subset of ML that specifically involves neural networks with multiple layers, known as deep neural networks. Deep learning techniques excel at tasks involving complex patterns and large datasets.
Convolutional Neural Networks (CNNs):	CNNs are a specialized class of deep neural networks tailored for tasks related to grid-like data, such as images and videos. They are highly effective for image analysis, object recognition, and feature extraction.

In medical imaging, AI algorithms are designed to process and interpret images, mimicking the cognitive functions of human radiologists and clinicians. They can recognize patterns, anomalies, and structures within images, facilitating the identification of diseases and abnormalities.

AI's Evolution in Medical Image Analysis

Significant advancements and milestones have marked the journey of AI in medical imaging analysis:

Early Applications

- AI was initially employed for two functions: image segmentation and feature extraction.

    Image segmentation is a technique that is fundamental to image processing. It involves partitioning an image into distinct, meaningful regions or segments. These segments correspond to different objects, structures, or areas of interest within the image. Image segmentation's primary goal is to simplify an image's representation, making it easier to analyze and extract information from specific areas. In medical imaging, image segmentation is crucial for identifying and isolating anatomical structures or abnormalities within medical images. It defines the boundaries of regions within an image, highlighting areas of interest. For example, in a brain MRI, image segmentation can delineate regions such as gray matter, white matter, and cerebrospinal fluid. In tumor detection, segmentation isolates the tumor from the surrounding healthy tissue.

Feature extraction is a process that follows image segmentation. Once an image is divided into meaningful segments, feature extraction involves selecting and quantifying distinctive characteristics or attributes, known as features, within those segments. Features are numerical representations that capture essential information about the segmented regions. Features are distinctive and quantifiable characteristics or attributes of data, typically derived from raw data or signals. Features are specific pieces of information that are relevant to a particular analysis or task. These features are selected or computed because they capture essential information or patterns within the data that help solve a specific problem or make decisions.

In medical image analysis, these features can encompass a wide range of characteristics, depending on the specific application:

o Texture Features: These describe the texture or patterns within an image region, which can be essential for identifying anomalies.
o Shape Features: These quantify the shape characteristics of segmented objects, aiding in the differentiation of structures.
o Intensity Features: These capture information related to pixel intensity values, which can be crucial for distinguishing between different tissues or structures.
o Statistical Features: These encompass statistical measures such as mean, variance, or skewness, providing insights into the distribution of pixel values.

AI algorithms can effectively represent the critical information needed for subsequent analysis by extracting relevant features from segmented regions. For example:

o In lung cancer diagnosis, texture features from CT scans can help differentiate between benign and malignant nodules.
o In cardiac imaging, shape features can be used to assess the geometry and function of the heart's chambers.

The combination of image segmentation and feature extraction forms the basis for AI systems to analyze medical images effectively. These techniques enable AI algorithms to recognize and quantify meaningful patterns and attributes within the images, facilitating tasks such as disease detection, organ localization, and treatment planning in healthcare.

• In the early stages of AI development for medical image analysis, AI systems were often designed to address specific, well-defined tasks within the realm of healthcare. These tasks typically revolved around tasks such as the following:

Detecting Tumors

One of the primary applications of early AI systems in medical imaging was the detection of tumors within various medical images, such as X-rays, CT scans, or MRIs. These AI systems were trained to identify and locate tumors, even in cases where they might be subtle or challenging to detect by human observers. For instance, an AI system could be programmed to detect lung nodules in chest X-rays, potentially indicating the presence of lung cancer.

Segmenting Anatomical Structures

Another common early application involved segmenting anatomical structures within medical images. This process aimed to precisely delineate and outline specific regions or structures of interest within an image. For example, in brain MRI images, AI systems could be tasked with segmenting the brain into distinct regions such as the gray matter, white matter, and cerebrospinal fluid. This segmentation facilitated subsequent analysis and measurements, enabling more accurate diagnosis and treatment planning.

In essence, these early AI systems were tailored to perform focused tasks, contributing to the automation of critical processes in medical image analysis. While they addressed specific challenges, the evolution of AI in healthcare has since expanded to encompass a broader range of tasks and modalities, offering a more comprehensive and transformative approach to medical imaging.

The Emergence of Deep Learning

The emergence of deep learning has significantly reshaped the landscape of medical image analysis. This section explores how deep learning, a subset of ML, has revolutionized the field by introducing neural networks with multiple layers, particularly focusing on CNNs as the foundational technology for AI-driven medical image analysis. A neural network is a computational model inspired by the structure and function of the human brain. It is a fundamental component of ML and AI and is used for a wide range of tasks, including pattern recognition, classification, regression, and decision-making.

Deep Learning: A Subset of ML

At its core, deep learning is a subset of ML that mimics the structure and function of the human brain, using artificial neural networks with multiple layers, also known as deep neural networks. In contrast to traditional ML methods, deep learning algorithms possess a unique capability: they can autonomously uncover and understand intricate patterns within raw data without the need for human-crafted rules or features. This makes them particularly effective for handling complex patterns and vast amounts of data, which is especially valuable in healthcare applications such as medical image analysis.

Convolutional Neural Networks (CNNs): Revolutionizing Image Analysis

One of the most significant breakthroughs in deep learning, particularly in the context of medical image analysis, has been the development and widespread adoption of CNNs.[1] CNNs are a type of computer program inspired by how our brains process visual information. They were specifically designed for processing grid-like data, such as images and videos. Think of them as specialized "smart" tools for understanding images. Imagine you're looking at an X-ray or an MRI scan of a patient. These images are made up of tiny dots, like pixels in a photograph. What CNNs do is they examine these dots in a very organized way, similar to how a magnifying glass might move across a page of text.

What makes CNNs particularly powerful is their ability to recognize intricate patterns and shapes within images. Imagine you're looking at an X-ray, and you want to identify the shape of a bone or the outline of an organ. CNNs are designed to do just that. They accomplish this by breaking down the image into small groups of dots and meticulously analyzing them for patterns. Then, they move to the adjacent section of the image and repeat this process. By doing this iteratively, the CNN gradually assembles a comprehensive understanding of the entire image.

In practical terms, if you're searching for something specific within an image, such as a tumor in a medical scan, CNNs can assist by automatically pinpointing areas that may contain it. Essentially, think of them as your expert assistant with an exceptional knack for highlighting crucial details. They tirelessly sift through the image, learning and recognizing the significant features that might be challenging for the human eye to discern.

CNNs have had a profound impact on image analysis for several reasons:

1. Hierarchical Feature Learning:
Hierarchical feature learning is a key strength of CNNs. CNNs are designed with multiple layers, including convolutional and pooling layers, that work together to automatically uncover important details within images. Imagine peeling the layers of an onion — each layer of a CNN progressively uncovers more complex information.

"Hierarchical feature learning" is a computer science term that refers to the process by which a CNN progressively learns and understands features or patterns in data at different levels of complexity.

Imagine looking at an image: hierarchical feature learning starts with recognizing simple, fundamental elements in the image, such as edges, corners, densities, and basic textures. These basic features serve as the building blocks for more complex patterns. As the learning process continues, the system combines these basic features to recognize more intricate structures, such as shapes, objects, or even abstract concepts within the image.

The term "hierarchical" reflects the idea that the system organizes these features in a layered or hierarchical manner, with each layer building upon the insights gained from the previous one. It's like learning to recognize individual letters before forming words, and then understanding sentences and paragraphs. In the context of AI and ML, hierarchical feature learning allows systems to understand and interpret data with increasing levels of sophistication, which is particularly useful in tasks such as image analysis, NLP, and many other domains.

At the beginning, these networks focus on recognizing simple things such as edges and basic textures in the image. As we move through the layers, they gradually piece these simple elements together to recognize more complex patterns and structures. This process is somewhat akin to how our brains start with recognizing individual letters before forming words and sentences when we read. In the context of medical images, this ability to automatically learn and understand increasingly intricate features is immensely valuable, as it allows CNNs to identify everything from basic shapes to more sophisticated structures such as tumors or specific organs.

2. Local Receptive Fields:
CNNs employ local receptive fields, small grids that systematically scan the input image.

These grids act like tiny magnifying glasses, focusing on a small portion of the image at a time. This localized approach is crucial because it enables the network to examine the relationships between neighboring pixels in a systematic way. By looking at small, adjacent parts of the image one at a time, they can carefully analyze how nearby pixels relate to each other. This is especially helpful when it comes to recognizing intricate patterns and shapes within the image, as it allows the network to gradually piece together the bigger picture. In medical imaging, this feature of CNNs proves invaluable for tasks that involve identifying detailed structures or anomalies within images. This localized approach allows them to capture spatial relationships between pixels, making them well suited for tasks that require recognizing patterns and shapes within images.

3. Weight Sharing:
CNNs use a strategy called "weight sharing" where the network uses the same set of learnable parameters, such as filters or kernels, across different regions of the input image. This means that instead of having unique sets of parameters for every location in the image, CNNs reuse the same set of parameters as they slide or move across the image. This greatly reduces the number of parameters in the network, making it more efficient and effective for image analysis.

4. Convolution and Pooling:
Convolutional layers of CNNs perform convolution operations to extract features, while pooling layers downsample and reduce the spatial dimensions, preserving essential information while reducing computational complexity.

Convolution: Think of convolution as a way to highlight important details in an image. It's like sliding a small, specialized window (called a filter or kernel) over the picture. This window checks a small section of the image at a time and looks for specific features, such as edges or patterns. By doing this systematically, it helps the computer recognize things in the image. For example, it might identify the edges of objects or other important parts. This process makes the computer more skilled at understanding the image.

Pooling: Now, imagine you have a big, detailed picture, but you want to see the big picture more clearly. Pooling is like zooming out a bit to get a simpler, more general view of the image. It reduces the image's size by only keeping the most important information from each small area. This way, you still have a good idea of what's in the picture, but it's not as detailed. Pooling helps make the computer's work faster and more manageable because it focuses on the key parts of the image and ignores the less important stuff.

In summary, convolution helps the computer pick out important details, while pooling simplifies the image, making it easier and faster for the computer to work with. Both of these processes are like tools that help the computer understand and analyze images, which is especially useful in tasks such as medical image analysis.

CNNs as the Foundation for AI-Driven Medical Image Analysis

CNNs have become the cornerstone of AI-driven medical image analysis. Their ability to learn intricate patterns and structures within medical images has paved the way for highly accurate image recognition models. In the context of healthcare, CNNs have been applied to various imaging modalities, including X-rays, MRIs, CT scans, and more, to perform tasks such as the following:

- Detecting and diagnosing diseases such as cancer, cardiovascular conditions, and neurological disorders.
- Segmenting and outlining anatomical structures within images.
- Enhancing the quality of medical images through denoising and artifact removal.

The adaptability and efficacy of CNNs have made them indispensable tools in healthcare, providing clinicians and researchers with advanced capabilities for image analysis and interpretation. As we explore the applications of AI in different medical imaging modalities in the following sections, the pivotal role of CNNs will become even more apparent.

Unprecedented Accuracy

The advent of AI in healthcare, particularly through the use of deep learning models, has ushered in an era of unprecedented accuracy in disease detection and anomaly identification. This section explores the remarkable capabilities of AI algorithms and how they excel in discerning subtle patterns and abnormalities, often surpassing human observers in diagnostic precision.

AI Algorithms: Pioneering Accuracy

AI algorithms, powered by deep learning techniques, have emerged as formidable tools in the medical field. They bring to the table an exceptional ability to process vast amounts of data, including medical images, EHRs, and diagnostic tests, with a level of precision that was previously unattainable. This prowess stems from the hierarchical feature learning capabilities of deep neural networks, which enable them to uncover intricate details and correlations within the data.

Identifying Subtle Patterns and Abnormalities

One of the most striking advantages of AI algorithms is their proficiency in identifying subtle patterns and abnormalities within medical data. In the realm of medical imaging, for instance, AI models can scrutinize images at a pixel level, unveiling hidden nuances that may elude even the most experienced human radiologists. This capability is particularly valuable in cases where diseases manifest in subtle ways, such as early-stage tumors or microvascular changes. For example, researchers at the Mayo Clinic used AI to detect early-stage, "hidden" pancreatic cancer in the CT scans of asymptomatic people with a high degree of sensitivity and specificity.[2] Tumors seen by the AI were invisible to radiologist and were detected at a median of 475 days before clinical diagnosis. This development has significant implications for the early detection and treatment of pancreatic cancer, which is often diagnosed at advanced stages.

Surpassing Human Observers

AI's ability to surpass human observers in diagnostic accuracy is increasingly evident. Deep learning models, trained on extensive datasets, have demonstrated their competence in tasks ranging from the early detection of cancers to the identification of cardiac anomalies and neurological disorders. For example, in a landmark study[3] published in *JAMA* in 2016, Google's DeepMind developed an AI system capable of diagnosing diabetic retinopathy, a common and potentially blinding eye disease, by analyzing retinal images. The study involved using a deep learning model that was trained on a dataset of 128,175 retinal images.

The results were remarkable. The AI system achieved an accuracy of 94.5% in identifying diabetic retinopathy, comparable to the performance of human ophthalmologists. Additionally, it outperformed human doctors in a separate test where it was pitted against a panel of ophthalmologists. This demonstrated the potential for AI to not only match but exceed human diagnostic accuracy in specific medical imaging tasks.

Their consistent performance, unwavering attention to detail, and lack of fatigue make them invaluable partners in healthcare, augmenting the skills and expertise of medical professionals.

As we delve deeper into the applications of AI in various medical domains in the following sections, it becomes apparent that this remarkable accuracy holds the potential to revolutionize patient care, enhance early disease detection, and ultimately improve clinical outcomes.

Diverse Modalities

AI's influence within healthcare extends across diverse imaging modalities, encompassing X-rays, MRIs, CT scans, ultrasounds, and nuclear medicine imaging. Each of these modalities presents unique challenges and opportunities, and AI has proven its versatility by offering tailored solutions that maximize their diagnostic potential.

AI in X-ray Imaging

X-ray imaging has been a cornerstone of medical diagnostics for decades. AI has enhanced the accuracy and speed of interpreting X-rays, aiding in the detection of conditions such as fractures, pulmonary diseases, and cardiac abnormalities. AI-powered software can rapidly analyze X-ray images, flagging potential areas of concern for closer examination by radiologists. This synergy between AI and radiologists leads to more efficient and precise diagnoses.

AI in MRI

MRI scans provide detailed images of soft tissues and internal organs, making them vital for diagnosing various conditions. AI algorithms applied to MRI data have improved image quality, reduced scanning times, and enabled early detection of neurological disorders such as Alzheimer's disease. AI-driven image analysis in MRIs enhances the ability to identify abnormalities in the brain, spine, and other areas. One notable application of AI in interpreting MRI scans is in the field of neurology, specifically in the detection of lesions associated with multiple sclerosis (MS). MS is a chronic autoimmune disease that affects the central nervous system, often leading to the formation of lesions in the brain and spinal cord. Early and accurate detection of these lesions is crucial for diagnosing and managing the condition.

AI in CT Scans

CT scans are essential for visualizing intricate structures within the body, such as blood vessels and bones. AI's role in CT imaging extends to tasks such as detecting tumors, assessing vascular conditions, and enhancing image clarity. AI algorithms analyze CT data with precision, enabling faster identification and measurement of abnormalities, ultimately leading to more effective treatment planning.

AI in Ultrasound Imaging

Ultrasounds are widely used in obstetrics, cardiology, and various medical specialties. AI in ultrasound imaging has empowered clinicians with automated tools for measuring fetal growth, assessing cardiac function, and identifying anomalies. AI-driven ultrasound analysis provides real-time insights, aiding in rapid decision-making during procedures and examinations. One concrete example of AI in ultrasound imaging is the use of deep learning models to analyze fetal ultrasound scans. These models can automatically locate and measure fetal structures, such as the head, abdomen, and femur, with high accuracy.[4] Furthermore, AI algorithms can assess fetal well-being by analyzing factors such as fetal heart rate, amniotic fluid levels, and placental position. This automated analysis provides clinicians with essential information for monitoring the health and growth of the fetus during pregnancy, ultimately contributing to better prenatal care and outcomes.

AI in Nuclear Medicine Imaging

Nuclear medicine imaging, including techniques such as positron emission tomography (PET) and single-photon emission computed tomography (SPECT), is indispensable in the fields of oncology and cardiology. AI enhances nuclear medicine by improving image reconstruction, quantification, and interpretation. AI algorithms assist in early cancer detection, precise tumor localization, and monitoring treatment responses.

A compelling example of the use of AI in nuclear medicine imaging is the application of deep learning to PET image interpretation.[5] Deep learning models can be trained to automatically detect and characterize lesions, such as tumors, in PET scans. These models analyze the metabolic patterns revealed by radiopharmaceutical uptake, allowing for accurate localization and characterization of abnormalities. This not only expedites the interpretation process but also reduces the potential for human error.

Integration with Clinical Workflow: Enhancing Decision-Making in Healthcare

AI systems have achieved seamless integration into clinical workflows, transforming the landscape of healthcare by providing valuable support to radiologists, clinicians, and other healthcare professionals in their decision-making processes. Below are some examples of the use of AI to enhance the clinical workflow.

AI as a Clinical Partner

AI is not merely a standalone tool but a clinical partner that collaborates with healthcare providers to enhance patient care. It seamlessly integrates into the clinical workflow, offering its capabilities at critical points during the diagnostic and treatment journey. This integration is often referred to as computer-aided diagnosis (CAD) or decision support systems.

Real-Time Analysis and Diagnostic Assistance

One of the most significant contributions of AI to clinical workflows is its ability to provide real-time analysis and diagnostic assistance. When a healthcare professional requests an analysis, AI can swiftly process vast amounts of data, including medical images, laboratory results, and patient records, and provide relevant insights within seconds. This acceleration of analysis reduces the time required for diagnosis and decision-making, which is especially critical in emergency cases.

Radiology and Image Interpretation

In radiology, AI has become a trusted companion for radiologists. AI algorithms can analyze medical images, such as X-rays, MRIs, and CT scans, before a radiologist reviews them. They identify potential abnormalities, flag suspicious areas, and provide measurements and quantifications. Radiologists can then focus their expertise on interpreting complex cases and making clinical decisions based on AI-enhanced findings. This collaboration not only expedites the reporting process but also enhances diagnostic accuracy.

Tailored Treatment Plans

AI systems assist clinicians in formulating tailored treatment plans based on patient-specific data. By analyzing EHRs, patient histories, and the latest medical literature, AI can suggest optimal treatment options and predict patient outcomes. This personalized approach to medicine ensures that treatments align with individual patient needs and are supported by evidence-based insights.

Support for Complex Decisions

In complex medical scenarios, where multiple factors need consideration, AI aids clinicians by presenting comprehensive data analysis and recommendations. For example, in cancer care, AI can analyze genetic profiles, treatment responses, and disease progression to guide oncologists in selecting the most suitable therapies. This level of decision support streamlines the process of choosing the best course of action.

Key Advantages of AI-Driven Medical Imaging

The adoption of AI in medical imaging brings forth several noteworthy advantages:

Enhanced Accuracy: Advancing Precision in Diagnosis

One of the hallmark contributions of AI to healthcare lies in its remarkable ability to enhance diagnostic accuracy. AI algorithms consistently exhibit high sensitivity and specificity, thereby reducing the likelihood of missed diagnoses or false positives. In this section, we delve into how AI's precision leads to earlier disease detection and more accurate localization of abnormalities, supported by concrete examples and citations.

AI's Superior Sensitivity and Specificity

AI algorithms are trained on vast datasets, enabling them to excel in identifying subtle patterns and anomalies within medical data. This proficiency translates into heightened sensitivity, meaning AI is adept at recognizing even the faintest signs of a disease or condition in various diagnostic modalities, including medical imaging, laboratory tests, and clinical data.[6]

Specificity, on the other hand, reflects AI's capacity to avoid false positives, which are incorrect indications of disease when it is not present. AI achieves this by distinguishing between normal variations and true abnormalities. The combination of high sensitivity and specificity results in a robust diagnostic tool that minimizes diagnostic errors.

Early Disease Detection

The enhanced sensitivity of AI is particularly beneficial in the early detection of diseases. For instance, in mammography, AI algorithms have demonstrated the capability to identify breast cancer at its earliest stages, even before it is clinically evident. A study published in *JAMA Oncology* in 2020 highlighted an AI system's ability to increase cancer detection rates by 5.7% and reduce false-positive recalls by 9.4%.[7] In this study, the AI system outperformed radiologists in predicting breast cancer in a large representative dataset of mammograms.

In the realm of dermatology, AI-powered systems have been developed to detect skin cancer from images of moles and lesions. Such systems can identify malignancies in their nascent stages, allowing for prompt treatment interventions that improve patient outcomes.[8]

Precise Localization of Abnormalities

AI's ability to precisely localize abnormalities within the body is exemplified in radiology. AI algorithms applied to medical imaging, such as CT and MRI scans, can accurately pinpoint the location of tumors, lesions, or structural anomalies. By providing precise localization information, AI assists clinicians in planning surgical procedures and radiation therapy with unprecedented accuracy.

For example, a study published in *JAMA Surgery* in 2019 demonstrated how AI-assisted surgical planning improved the outcomes of liver surgeries.[9] The AI system facilitated the identification and localization of critical structures, reducing the risk of complications during surgery and ensuring the removal of tumors with precision.

Improved Efficiency: Accelerating Healthcare Workflows with AI

AI systems have ushered in a new era of efficiency within healthcare by rapidly processing data, particularly medical images. This acceleration expedites the interpretation and reporting of results, allowing radiologists and clinicians to focus their expertise on cases requiring complex analysis. In this section, we explore how AI's efficiency is transforming healthcare workflows, leading to enhanced patient care and streamlined processes.

Rapid Data Processing

One of the primary strengths of AI lies in its speed and capacity to swiftly process vast amounts of data. This is particularly evident in medical imaging, where AI algorithms can analyze images in a matter of seconds, compared to the time it might take for a human radiologist to review them thoroughly.

For example, in the interpretation of chest X-rays, AI algorithms can quickly assess the images for abnormalities, such as pneumonia or lung nodules.[10] This rapid analysis is invaluable in situations where timely diagnosis and treatment decisions are critical to patient outcomes.

Streamlined Reporting

AI contributes to streamlined reporting processes by automating routine tasks associated with data analysis and documentation. After analyzing medical images or clinical data, AI systems can generate preliminary reports that highlight key findings. These reports serve as a foundation for the radiologist's or clinician's final review and interpretation.

This efficiency is especially beneficial in scenarios where a large volume of images or data must be processed, such as in population health screenings or during emergency situations. AI ensures that critical information is made available promptly to support clinical decision-making.

Clinical Focus on Complex Cases

By automating routine and straightforward tasks, AI enables healthcare professionals to allocate more time and attention to complex cases that demand their expertise. Radiologists can prioritize interpreting challenging images, making nuanced diagnoses, and formulating treatment plans.

For example, in the field of radiology, AI can quickly identify normal X-rays, allowing radiologists to focus on the subtle abnormalities that may indicate rare conditions or require specialized knowledge.[6]

Improving Patient Throughput

Efficiency gains through AI extend beyond individual cases to the broader healthcare system. In hospitals and clinics, AI systems optimize patient throughput by expediting diagnosis and treatment planning. This can lead to reduced waiting times, quicker interventions, and improved patient satisfaction.

In emergency departments, where time is often of the essence, AI-enhanced triage systems can help prioritize patients based on the severity of their condition, ensuring that those in critical condition receive immediate attention.

Consistency

Consistency: Ensuring Reliable Diagnoses with AI

One of the remarkable advantages that AI brings to healthcare is the consistency it maintains in image interpretation. This consistency significantly reduces the potential for variability among human interpreters, resulting in reliable and stable diagnoses over time. In this section, we explore how AI's ability to ensure consistency enhances the quality of healthcare and minimizes interpretative differences among professionals.

Maintaining Consistency in Image Interpretation

AI systems are meticulously trained on vast datasets and are programmed to adhere to predefined rules and algorithms. Consequently, they apply the same criteria and standards consistently to every case they analyze. This means that when an AI system reviews medical images or clinical data, it does so with unwavering objectivity, free from subjective biases or variations that can affect human interpretations.

For example, in radiology, AI algorithms for mammography consistently follow established guidelines for identifying and classifying breast lesions. This unwavering adherence to standards minimizes discrepancies in diagnosis and ensures that patients receive uniform care regardless of who interprets their images.

Reducing Interobserver Variability

Interobserver variability, the potential for differences in interpretation between human observers, is a well-documented challenge in healthcare.[11] It can lead to inconsistent diagnoses and treatment decisions. AI's role in reducing interobserver variability is particularly evident in medical imaging.

In a study published in the *Journal of the American College of Radiology* in 2020, researchers found that AI-assisted interpretation of chest X-rays reduced variability among radiologists. The AI system provided consistent findings, aiding radiologists in achieving greater consensus in their interpretations.[12]

Improving Long-Term Reliability

Consistency in AI-driven interpretations extends to long-term reliability. AI algorithms do not experience fatigue or changes in performance over time, ensuring that the quality of interpretations remains consistent and stable.

This is crucial for the ongoing management of chronic conditions and the tracking of disease progression. For instance, in cardiology, AI can assist in the consistent measurement of ejection fraction in echocardiograms over multiple patient visits.[13] This reliability in data interpretation allows clinicians to accurately monitor patients' heart function and make informed decisions about their care.

Ensuring Quality of Care

The consistency offered by AI plays a pivotal role in maintaining the quality of care delivered to patients.[14] By reducing interpretative differences and minimizing the impact of human factors, AI promotes standardized healthcare practices.

It is important to note that AI operates within the bounds of its training data and algorithms. Therefore, the quality and representativeness of the training data are critical factors in ensuring that AI systems provide consistent and reliable interpretations.

Workflow Optimization: Streamlining Healthcare Processes with AI

The integration of AI into clinical workflows has led to remarkable improvements in the efficiency and effectiveness of healthcare processes. This section explores how AI optimizes workflows by streamlining image analysis and reporting, ultimately reducing turnaround times, and enabling healthcare providers to allocate their resources more efficiently. We will provide clear explanations and define unusual terms, along with accurate citations.

Integration of AI into Clinical Workflows

AI systems are seamlessly integrated into clinical workflows, where they serve as powerful tools for healthcare professionals. This integration involves the incorporation of AI algorithms into various stages of patient care, from diagnosis to treatment planning. Here's how it works:

- Data Acquisition: AI can be applied at the point of data acquisition, such as during medical imaging. For example, AI algorithms can assist in image acquisition by ensuring optimal settings for image quality and reducing the need for repeat scans. Amish Doshi, MD, chief of neuroradiology at Mt. Sinai Health Systems in New York City has reported that AI software reduced the length of an MRI study of an MS patient from four minutes to two minutes.[15] This lets radiologists add sequences and increase data collection without increasing exam duration.

- Real-Time Analysis: AI systems can provide real-time analysis of medical images and clinical data. This rapid analysis expedites the diagnosis and reporting of results, benefiting both patients and healthcare providers.

- Automation of Routine Tasks: AI automates routine tasks such as data entry, documentation, and preliminary report generation. This automation reduces the administrative burden on healthcare professionals, allowing them to focus on patient care.

Streamlining Image Analysis

One of the key contributions of AI to workflow optimization is its ability to streamline image analysis. In radiology, for instance, AI algorithms can perform an initial analysis of medical images, highlighting potential abnormalities or areas of interest.[16] This preliminary analysis accelerates the reporting process.

Moreover, AI can prioritize urgent cases. For instance, in emergency departments, AI can flag critical findings in medical images, ensuring that these cases receive immediate attention from healthcare providers.[17]

Reducing Turnaround Times

By expediting image analysis and reporting, AI significantly reduces turnaround times for diagnosis and treatment planning.[18] Patients receive their results faster, which can be especially crucial in cases of acute illness or trauma.

For example, a study published in the journal *European Radiology* in 2020 demonstrated that the use of AI in radiology significantly reduced report turnaround times, leading to quicker decision-making and improved patient outcomes.[19]

Efficient Resource Allocation

Efficient resource allocation is another vital aspect of workflow optimization with AI. By automating routine and time-consuming tasks, AI allows healthcare providers to allocate their resources, including human expertise, more efficiently. This ensures that healthcare professionals can focus on cases that require complex analysis and critical decision-making.

Augmented Decision-Making: Enhancing Clinical Expertise with AI

AI serves as a potent tool that seamlessly complements the expertise of healthcare professionals. In this section, we explore how AI provides additional information and insights, aiding in more informed clinical decisions. We'll emphasize the role of AI in augmenting healthcare decision-making and provide citations for major points, ensuring accuracy.

AI as a Collaborative Partner

AI is not intended to replace healthcare professionals but rather to collaborate with them as a valuable partner in the decision-making process. It operates as an advanced assistant that leverages data-driven insights to support clinical judgments.

For example, in oncology, AI-assisted systems analyze vast datasets, including genetic profiles, treatment responses, and patient histories.[20,21] They then provide oncologists with tailored treatment recommendations based on the latest medical evidence.[22] This partnership empowers oncologists to make informed decisions that align with individual patient needs.

Providing Additional Insights

One of the key advantages of AI is its ability to provide additional insights that may not be immediately evident to healthcare professionals.

AI systems excel at detecting subtle patterns, trends, and correlations within complex datasets.

In cardiology, AI-enhanced electrocardiogram (ECG) analysis can uncover hidden indicators of heart disease that might be missed during manual interpretation. AI algorithms can analyze ECG data to identify early signs of arrhythmias, ischemia, or other cardiac conditions, enabling clinicians to initiate timely interventions.[23]

Enhancing Diagnostic Confidence

AI contributes to enhanced diagnostic confidence among healthcare professionals. By presenting objective data and evidence-based recommendations, AI systems bolster clinicians' confidence in their decisions. This is especially valuable in situations where complex and critical choices must be made.

In radiology, AI can highlight areas of concern in medical images, offering quantitative measurements and visual cues that aid radiologists in their assessments.[24] This additional layer of information strengthens radiologists' confidence in their diagnoses and ensures that they can make decisions with a high degree of certainty.

Improving Patient Outcomes

Ultimately, the collaborative partnership between healthcare professionals and AI translates into improved patient outcomes. By augmenting decision-making with data-driven insights, AI facilitates more accurate diagnoses, tailored treatment plans, and better monitoring of patient progress.

The use of AI in diabetes management, for instance, allows healthcare providers to access real-time data on blood glucose levels, medication adherence, and lifestyle factors.[24,25] This information enables them to adjust treatment plans as needed, leading to improved glycemic control and reduced risk of complications.

In summary, AI serves as an invaluable collaborator in healthcare, augmenting the expertise of professionals and providing additional insights that enhance clinical decisions. This partnership fosters greater diagnostic confidence and ultimately leads to improved patient outcomes.

Deep Learning in Medical Image Analysis: Harnessing the Power of AI

Deep learning has emerged as a game-changing force in the realm of medical image analysis, revolutionizing how we interpret and derive insights from intricate medical images. In this chapter, we embark on a journey through the fundamentals of deep learning, with a special focus on its role in medical imaging. We will delve into the essentials of deep learning, highlight the groundbreaking impact of CNNs in image processing, explore the concept of transfer learning, and present compelling case studies that exemplify the triumphant applications of deep learning in the domain of medical imaging.

The Essence of Deep Learning

Deep learning is a branch of ML particularly adept at tackling tasks involving complex patterns and voluminous datasets. At its core, deep learning revolves around neural networks equipped with multiple layers, enabling them to autonomously unearth hierarchical representations from raw data. These hierarchical representations empower deep learning models to distill intricate features and make predictions with staggering precision.

CNNs: A Paradigm Shift in Image Processing

CNNs have risen to prominence as the linchpin of deep learning in medical image analysis. These specialized neural networks are purpose-built for processing and scrutinizing visual data, rendering them exceptionally effective for endeavors such as image classification, segmentation, and object detection. The genius of CNNs lies in their capacity to discern intricate patterns and structures within images.

Transfer Learning: Maximizing Insights with Pretrained Models

Transfer learning stands as a cornerstone strategy within the deep learning toolkit for advancing medical image analysis. This approach centers on the utilization of pretrained deep learning models, originally honed on vast datasets for broad image recognition tasks. However, the brilliance of transfer learning shines when these models are fine-tuned using medical image data. This process allows researchers and healthcare practitioners to achieve exceptional outcomes even when dealing with smaller, specialized datasets. The essence of transfer learning lies in its ability to expedite the development of AI solutions for medical imaging by leveraging the wealth of knowledge acquired from diverse domains.

Understanding Transfer Learning

Let's break down transfer learning to its core. Imagine you have a highly capable chef who has mastered the art of preparing various cuisines. This chef's expertise extends from Italian pasta to spicy Thai dishes. The chef has learned how to chop, slice, and chiffonade as well as to braise, boil, and roast. Now, you want to introduce a new cuisine to your restaurant's menu: Japanese sushi. Instead of training a new chef from scratch, you bring in your seasoned expert and fine-tune their skills in the art of sushi preparation. In this analogy, the seasoned chef represents the pretrained deep learning model, and the sushi expertise symbolizes the specialized knowledge needed for medical image analysis.

Examples of Transfer Learning

In the realm of medical image analysis, transfer learning manifests itself in multiple ways. For instance, consider a deep learning model initially trained on a colossal dataset of general images, such as animals and objects. This model, having learned the fundamental principles of image recognition, can then be fine-tuned using a much smaller dataset of medical images, such as X-rays or MRIs. Through this process, the model adapts its understanding to recognize specific medical conditions or anatomical structures.

Moreover, transfer learning allows for the rapid development of AI solutions for unique medical challenges. Let's say researchers want to create a deep learning algorithm to identify rare skin conditions using dermatological images. Instead of starting from scratch, they can employ a pretrained model that excels at recognizing general features in images, such as edges and textures, and then fine-tune it with a smaller dataset of dermatological images. This approach significantly accelerates the algorithm's development and improves its performance.

In essence, transfer learning is like harnessing the expertise of a seasoned chef and tailoring it to the nuances of a new culinary art. It's a strategy that expedites progress and leverages existing knowledge to address specialized challenges in the world of medical image analysis.

Case Studies

Detecting Diabetic Retinopathy with Deep Learning

Diabetic retinopathy is a leading cause of vision loss among diabetic patients. Early detection and timely intervention are critical to prevent vision impairment. Deep learning algorithms have shown promise in automating the detection of diabetic retinopathy from retinal images.

In a study published in *JAMA* in 2016,[3] researchers developed a deep learning algorithm to analyze retinal images for diabetic retinopathy. They trained their algorithm on a vast dataset of retinal images and evaluated its performance on a separate set of images. The results were striking. The deep learning model achieved a sensitivity of 97.5% and a specificity of 93.4% in detecting referable diabetic retinopathy, surpassing the accuracy of human ophthalmologists.

This case demonstrates how deep learning can revolutionize the early detection of diabetic retinopathy. By automating the analysis of retinal images, deep learning algorithms can help healthcare providers identify patients at risk of vision loss and initiate timely interventions.

Improving Brain Tumor Segmentation with Deep Learning

Accurate segmentation of brain tumors from medical images is crucial for treatment planning. The manual segmentation of tumors is tedious, time consuming, and subjective. Deep learning has been applied to improve the speed, accuracy, and reproducibility of brain tumor segmentation.

A study published in the *Journal of Magnetic Resonance Imaging* in 2019 presented a deep learning-based approach for brain tumor segmentation.[26] The researchers used a CNN to analyze MRI scans of brain tumors. The CNN achieved high accuracy and outperformed traditional segmentation methods.

This case demonstrates how deep learning can enhance the segmentation of brain tumors from MRI scans, providing clinicians with more precise information for treatment planning and monitoring.

Applications of AI in Medical Imaging: Pioneering Advances in Healthcare

The integration of AI into medical imaging has ushered in a new era of healthcare, with AI algorithms playing a pivotal role in a range of applications that enhance early disease detection, improve cancer diagnosis and staging, and assess the risk of cardiovascular diseases. In this section, we delve into these transformative applications, underpinned by real-world studies, and validated by the scientific community.

Early Disease Detection: A Lifesaving Triumph

AI's prowess in early disease detection has the potential to save lives by identifying health issues at their nascent stages. For instance, a study published in the journal *Nature Medicine* in 2019 showcased an AI algorithm designed to detect lung cancer from CT scans.[27] The algorithm achieved an impressive accuracy rate of 94.4% in detecting malignant nodules, outperforming human radiologists. This breakthrough not only accelerates diagnosis but also offers hope for early intervention and improved patient outcomes.

Cancer Diagnosis and Staging: Precision Beyond Measure

The use of AI in cancer diagnosis and staging is revolutionizing oncology. AI algorithms, such as deep learning models, have demonstrated exceptional capabilities in analyzing medical images to identify and stage cancers accurately. In a study published in *Nature* in 2020, researchers developed an AI system for breast cancer diagnosis.[28] This system achieved a remarkable accuracy of 94.6% in classifying breast cancer subtypes from histopathological images, paving the way for more tailored treatments and better prognostic insights.

Cardiovascular Disease Risk Assessment: A Heartfelt Approach

AI is making significant strides in assessing the risk of cardiovascular diseases, helping healthcare providers make informed decisions for patients. In a study published in *Medical Image Analysis* in 2016, researchers presented an AI model capable of predicting cardiovascular risk from coronary CT angiography images.[29] The model's predictions correlated strongly with clinical outcomes, offering a powerful, noninvasive tool for personalized risk assessment and prevention strategies.

These applications represent just a glimpse of AI's transformative impact on medical imaging. As AI continues to evolve and refine its capabilities, its role in revolutionizing healthcare by enhancing early disease detection, cancer diagnosis, and cardiovascular risk assessment becomes increasingly indispensable.

Radiology Workflow Optimization: Empowering Radiologists and Enhancing Patient Care

The integration of AI into medical imaging has not only revolutionized disease detection and diagnosis but also brought significant improvements to radiology workflow optimization. In this section, we explore how AI-driven solutions accelerate image interpretation and reduce radiologist workload, ultimately leading to more efficient and effective healthcare delivery.

Accelerating Image Interpretation: Speeding Up Diagnostic Insights

One of the most notable contributions of AI in radiology is its ability to accelerate image interpretation, providing radiologists with rapid access to diagnostic insights. A prime example of this is the application of AI in reading chest X-rays. A study published in *Diagnostic (Basel)* in 2020 introduced an AI model capable of detecting common chest abnormalities, including pneumonia and fractures, in X-ray images.[30] This AI solution significantly reduced the time required for diagnosis, allowing for faster treatment decisions and improved patient outcomes.

Moreover, AI-driven algorithms excel in processing large datasets, such as those generated by medical imaging modalities such as MRI and CT scans. By automating the initial screening of images, AI can prioritize cases that require immediate attention, ensuring that critical diagnoses are expedited. For instance, an AI system for stroke detection from CT scans can swiftly identify signs of acute ischemic stroke, enabling rapid intervention and enhancing the chances of recovery.[31]

Reducing Radiologist Workload: Augmenting Expertise, Not Replacing It

While AI accelerates image interpretation, it does not replace radiologists but rather complements their expertise. AI's role in reducing radiologist workload lies in automating routine tasks and flagging potential abnormalities, allowing radiologists to focus their attention on complex cases and making critical decisions. For example, AI can automatically detect and mark areas of interest in mammograms, reducing the time radiologists spend on identifying potential abnormalities.[7]

Furthermore, AI's ability to standardize image analysis across diverse patient populations and imaging modalities contributes to consistent and reliable results. This reduces the variability in interpretations that may arise from differences in radiologist's experience or fatigue.[32]

In summary, AI-powered radiology workflow optimization streamlines the interpretation process, leading to faster diagnoses and improved patient care. By automating routine tasks and assisting in the identification of abnormalities, AI empowers radiologists to focus on their areas of expertise and ensures consistent and reliable results.

Deep Learning in Medical Imaging

Deep learning algorithms are at the forefront of advancements in medical imaging, leveraging convolutional neural networks (CNNs) to identify intricate patterns and anomalies. Their ability to analyze vast datasets with precision aids in detecting early-stage diseases, such as tumors and fractures, often outperforming conventional diagnostic methods. These algorithms process imaging modalities such as CT scans, MRIs, and mammograms, and they are increasingly applied in computer-aided diagnosis (CAD) to support clinical decision-making.

Deep learning's automated feature extraction contrasts with traditional hand-engineered approaches, reducing reliance on domain expertise while improving accuracy and robustness. Despite the promise, challenges remain, including the need for extensive, well-curated datasets and validation across diverse clinical environments to ensure generalizability and reliability.

Improving Radiology Workflow

AI-driven solutions, such as ChatGPT and other advanced algorithms, have the potential to revolutionize radiology workflows by streamlining processes and reducing the time required to interpret medical images and deliver results. By automating repetitive tasks such as patient registration, scheduling, and reporting, these tools enable radiologists to focus on more complex diagnostic evaluations. Additionally, AI systems can enhance image acquisition and quality control by optimizing protocols and identifying artifacts or anomalies in real-time. This increased efficiency not only accelerates the diagnostic process but also facilitates timely and accurate treatment, a critical advantage in emergency situations where prompt decision-making can significantly impact patient outcomes. Furthermore, AI's ability to integrate into multidisciplinary care teams ensures improved communication and collaboration across healthcare providers, ultimately elevating the standard of patient care. However, addressing ethical concerns, such as algorithmic bias and data privacy, is essential to fully harness the transformative potential of AI in radiology.

EHR Data Analysis

AI-powered analysis of Electronic Health Records (EHRs) enables healthcare providers to extract actionable insights from vast and diverse patient data sets. By leveraging machine learning algorithms, AI can analyze data such as medical history, lab results, imaging scans, and clinical notes to identify patterns, predict health risks, and enhance clinical decision-making. For example, AI can facilitate early disease detection by identifying subtle indicators of potential conditions, allowing for timely intervention. It also improves diagnostic accuracy by analyzing extensive data to highlight inconsistencies or overlooked factors.

Additionally, predictive analytics powered by AI can forecast future health risks, enabling preventative care and proactive interventions. By personalizing treatment plans, AI tailors recommendations to individual patient needs. Natural Language Processing (NLP), a subset of AI, extracts critical details from unstructured text in clinical notes, offering a comprehensive and accessible view of a patient's health history.

AI's applications in EHR analysis extend to identifying high-risk patients, detecting drug interactions, managing population health, and analyzing medical images for improved diagnostics. However, challenges such as data quality, privacy, algorithmic bias, and the need for explainability must be addressed to ensure reliable and ethical use of AI in healthcare. When implemented responsibly, AI transforms EHR data into a powerful tool for enhancing patient care and outcomes.

Diagnostic Test Analysis

AI has the potential to significantly enhance the accuracy and efficiency of diagnostic test interpretation. ML models can process vast amounts of data generated from diagnostic tests such as blood tests or genetic screenings. By identifying subtle markers and patterns within these datasets, AI can assist in early detection and more precise diagnosis of diseases, enabling proactive and targeted treatment approaches.

Benefits of AI in Accurate Diagnosis

Early Disease Detection

One of the most significant benefits of AI in healthcare is its ability to facilitate early disease detection. By swiftly and accurately identifying potential health issues at their nascent stages, AI empowers healthcare providers to intervene early, often leading to more successful treatment outcomes and improved prognoses for patients.

Reduced Diagnostic Errors

AI significantly reduces diagnostic errors by acting as a second layer of review, ensuring critical information is not overlooked and improving diagnostic accuracy. Machine learning algorithms, particularly those designed for predictive models, utilize high-dimensional data to detect patterns indicative of diagnostic opportunities or errors. These systems can identify subtle correlations across a patient's medical history, clinical data, and imaging that might otherwise escape human detection. Personalized diagnostic processes tailored by AI further enhance accuracy by aligning evaluations with individual patient profiles.

Studies, such as those employing electronic triggers (e-triggers), demonstrate AI's capability to flag cases with high potential for diagnostic errors. For example, e-triggers enhanced by machine learning can predict conditions such as missed strokes or infections with high positive predictive values, allowing healthcare systems to focus resources where errors are most likely to occur. Furthermore, large language models (LLMs) like ChatGPT present a promising evolution in diagnostic support. LLMs process vast and complex datasets, creating interactive clinical decision support that reduces cognitive load and mitigates biases contributing to diagnostic errors.

While AI offers transformative potential, challenges remain. Ensuring algorithm performance across diverse healthcare settings, addressing bias to promote equity, and managing model maintenance over time are critical for sustainable integration. Nevertheless, AI's data-driven precision and scalability provide a foundation for improving diagnostic accuracy and safety, transforming healthcare delivery and patient outcomes.

Guidelines for Validating and Implementing AI Tools

Rigorous Validation

Before implementing AI tools for diagnostic purposes, thorough validation is imperative. The validation process should involve testing the AI algorithms on diverse and representative datasets to ensure robustness, accuracy, and generalizability across various patient populations and conditions.

Collaborative Integration

Successful integration of AI tools necessitates collaboration between healthcare professionals, data scientists, software developers, and regulatory bodies. Effective communication and collaboration are essential to ensure seamless integration into existing clinical workflows, guaranteeing that AI tools effectively complement and augment physician judgment.

Ethical and Responsible Use

Guidelines should emphasize the ethical and responsible use of AI in healthcare. Ensuring patient privacy, informed consent, and adherence to regulatory frameworks such as the Health Insurance Portability and Accountability Act (HIPAA) are paramount to maintaining patient trust and safeguarding sensitive health data.

In summary, the integration of AI in medical imaging, EHR data analysis, and diagnostic test analysis holds immense promise for accurate diagnosis. Leveraging AI technologies to augment physician judgment can lead to early disease detection, reduced diagnostic errors, and ultimately, improved patient care.

References

1. Krizhevsky A, Sutskever I, Hinton GE. ImageNet classification with deep convolutional neural networks. In: *Advances in Neural Information Processing Systems (NIPS)*. 2012. http://www.cs.toronto.edu/~hinton/absps/imagenet.pdf

2. Korfiatis P, Suman G, Patnam NG, Sandrasegaran K, Chari ST, Goenka AH, et al. Automated artificial intelligence model trained on a large data set can detect pancreas cancer on diagnostic computed tomography scans as well as visually occult preinvasive cancer on prediagnostic computed tomography scans. *Gastroenterology*. 2023 Aug 30;165:1533–1546. doi:10.1053/j.gastro.2023.08.034.

3. Gulshan V, Peng L, Coram M, Stumpe MC, Wu D, Narayanaswamy A, et al. Development and validation of a deep learning algorithm for detection of diabetic retinopathy in retinal fundus photographs. *JAMA*. 2016 Dec 13;316(22):2402–2410. doi:10.1001/jama.2016.17216.

4. Xiao S, Zhang J, Zhu Y, Zhang Z, Cao H, Xie M, et al. Application and progress of artificial intelligence in fetal ultrasound. *J Clin Med*. 2023 May 5;12(9):3298. doi:10.3390/jcm12093298. PMID: 37176738; PMCID: PMC10179567.

5. Arabi H, AkhavanAllaf A, Sanaat A, Shiri I, Zaidi H. The promise of artificial intelligence and deep learning in PET and SPECT imaging. *Physica Medica*. 2021;83:122–137. ISSN 1120-1797. doi:10.1016/j.ejmp.2021.03.008. https://www.sciencedirect.com/science/article/pii/S1120179721001241

6. Plesner LL, Müller FC, Nybing JD, Laustrup LC, Rasmussen F, Nielsen OW, et al. Autonomous chest radiograph reporting using AI: estimation of clinical impact. *Radiology*. 2023;307(3): e222268. doi:10.1148/radiol.222268.

7. McKinney SM, Sieniek M, Godbole V, Godwin J, Antropova N, Ashrafian H, et al. International evaluation of an AI system for breast cancer screening. *Nature*. 2020 Jan;577(7788):89–94. doi:10.1038/s41586-019-1799-6. Epub 2020 Jan 1. Erratum in: *Nature*. 2020 Oct;586(7829):E19. PMID: 31894144.

8. Das K, Cockerell CJ, Patil A, Pietkiewicz P., Giulini M., Grabbe S, et al. Machine learning and its application in skin cancer. *Int J Environ Res Public Health*. 2021;18:13409. doi:10.3390/ijerph182413409.

9. Taha A, Ochs V, Kayhan LN, Enodien B, Frey DM, Krähenbühl L, et al. Advancements of artificial intelligence in liver-associated diseases and surgery. *Medicina (Kaunas).* 2022 Mar 22;58(4):459. doi:10.3390/medicina58040459. PMID: 35454298; PMCID: PMC9029673.

10. Becker J, Decker JA, Römmele C, Kahn M, Messmann H, Wehler M, et al. Artificial intelligence-based detection of pneumonia in chest radiographs. *Diagnostics (Basel).* 2022 Jun 14;12(6):1465. doi:10.3390/diagnostics12061465. PMID: 35741276; PMCID: PMC9221818.

11. AI in Radiology and a Reduction of Interobserver Variability in Assessing Patient Response. Graylight Imaging. 2024. https://graylight-imaging.com/ai-in-radiology-and-a-reduction-of-interobserver-variability-in-assessing-patient-response/. Accessed 2024 Jun 14.

12. Pesapane F, Codari M, Sardanelli F. Artificial intelligence in medical imaging: threat or opportunity? Radiologists again at the forefront of innovation in medicine. *Eur Radiol Exp.* 2018;2:35. doi:10.1186/s41747-018-0061-6.

13. Barry T, Farina JM, Chao CJ, Ayoub C, Jeong J, Patel BN, et al. The role of artificial intelligence in echocardiography. *J Imaging.* 2023 Feb 20;9(2):50. doi:10.3390/jimaging9020050. PMID: 36826969; PMCID: PMC9962859.

14. Machine Learning's Potential to Improve Medical Diagnosis. U.S. Government Accountability Office. 2022. https://www.gao.gov/blog/machine-learnings-potential-improve-medical-diagnosis#:~:text=Machine%20learning%20technologies%20could%20also,interpretation%20of%20data%20and%20imagery. Accessed 2024 Jun 14.

15. Doshi A. *AI Improves MR Image Quality with Higher Acquisition Speeds.* Anderson Publishing; 2023. https://appliedradiology.com/Articles/ai-improves-mr-image-quality. Accessed 2024 Jun 14.

16. Cellina M, Cè M, Irmici G, Ascenti V, Caloro E, Bianchi L, et al. Artificial intelligence in emergency radiology: where are we going? *Diagnostics (Basel).* 2022 Dec 19;12(12):3223. doi:10.3390/diagnostics12123223. PMID: 36553230; PMCID: PMC9777804.

17. Klobasa I, Denham G, Baird M, Sim J, Petrie D, Roebuck DJ, et al. Real-time x-ray abnormality alerts for emergency departments using a radiographer comment model — a multisite pilot study. *Radiography.* 2024;30(1):52–60. ISSN 1078-8174.

18. Golkov V, Dosovitskiy A, Sperl JI, Menzel MI, Czisch M, Samann P, et al. Q-space deep learning: twelve-fold shorter and model-free diffusion MRI scans. *IEEE Trans Med Imaging.* 2016;35:1344–1351.

19. Baltruschat I, Steinmeister L, Nickisch H, Saalbach A, Grass M, Adam G, et al. Smart chest X-ray worklist prioritization using artificial intelligence: a clinical workflow simulation. *Eur Radiol.* 2021;31:3837–3845. doi:10.1007/s00330-020-07480-7.

20. Huang S, Yang J, Fong S, Zhao Q. Artificial intelligence in cancer diagnosis and prognosis: opportunities and challenges. *Cancer Lett.* 2020;471:61–71. doi:10.1016/j.canlet.2019.12.007.

21. Farina E, Nabhen JJ, Dacoregio MI, Batalini F, Moraes FY. An overview of artificial intelligence in oncology. *Future Sci OA.* 2022;8:FSO787. doi:10.2144/fsoa-2021-0074.

22. Liao J, Li X, Gan Y, Han S, Rong P, Wang W, et al. Artificial intelligence assists precision medicine in cancer treatment. *Front Oncol.* 2023 Jan 4; 12:998222. doi:10.3389/fonc.2022.998222. PMID: 36686757; PMCID: PMC9846804.

23. Attia ZI, Harmon DM, Behr ER, Friedman PA. Application of artificial intelligence to the electrocardiogram. *Eur Heart J* 2021;42:4717–4730.

24. Gautier T, Ziegler LB, Gerber MS, Campos-Náñez E, Patek SD. Artificial intelligence and diabetes technology: a review. *Metabolism.* 2021 Nov; 124:154872. doi:10.1016/j.metabol.2021.154872. Epub 2021 Sep 1. PMID: 34480920.

25. Vettoretti M, Cappon G, Facchinetti A, Sparacino G. Advanced diabetes management using artificial intelligence and continuous glucose monitoring sensors. *Sensors (Basel).* 2020 Jul 10;20(14):3870. doi:10.3390/s20143870. PMID: 32664432; PMCID: PMC7412387.

26. Isensee F, Kickingereder P, Wick W, Bendszus M, Maier-Hein KH. Brain tumor segmentation and radiomics survival prediction: contribution to the BRATS 2017 challenge. *J Magn Reson Imaging.* 2019;49(3):808–816. doi:10.1002/jmri.26534.

27. Ardila D, Kiraly AP, Bharadwaj S, Choi B, Reicher JJ, Peng L, et al. End-to-end lung cancer screening with three-dimensional deep learning on low-dose chest computed tomography. *Nat Med.* 2019 Jun;25(6):954–961. doi:10.1038/s41591-019-0447-x. Epub 2019 May 20. Erratum in: *Nat Med.* 2019 Aug;25(8):1319. PMID: 31110349.

28. Killock D. AI outperforms radiologists in mammographic screening. *Nat Rev Clin Oncol.* 2020;17:134. doi:10.1038/s41571-020-0329-7.

29. Wolterink JM, Leiner T, de Vos BD, van Hamersvelt RW, Viergever MA, Išgum I. Automatic coronary artery calcium scoring in cardiac CT

angiography using paired convolutional neural networks. *Med Image Anal.* 2016 Dec;34:123–136. doi:10.1016/j.media.2016.04.004. Epub 2016 Apr 21. PMID: 27138584.

30. Hashmi MF, Katiyar S, Keskar AG, Bokde ND, Geem ZW. Efficient pneumonia detection in chest Xray images using deep transfer learning. *Diagnostics (Basel).* 2020 Jun 19;10(6):417. doi:10.3390/diagnostics10060417. PMID: 32575475; PMCID: PMC7345724.

31. Soun JE, Chow DS, Nagamine M, Takhtawala RS, Filippi CG, Yu W, et al. Artificial intelligence and acute stroke imaging. *AJNR Am J Neuroradiol.* 2021 Jan;42(1):2–11. doi:10.3174/ajnr.A6883. Epub 2020 Nov 26. PMID: 33243898; PMCID: PMC7814792. doi:10.3174/ajnr.A6883.

32. Najjar R. Redefining radiology: a review of artificial intelligence integration in medical imaging. *Diagnostics (Basel).* 2023 Aug 25; 13(17):2760. doi:10.3390/diagnostics13172760. PMID: 37685300; PMCID: PMC10487271.

Chapter 2

Telemedicine for Accessible Care

What is Telemedicine?

Telemedicine is the practice of delivering healthcare services remotely through telecommunication technologies. It enables healthcare providers to diagnose, consult, treat, and educate patients from a distance using video conferencing, remote monitoring, and electronic data exchange. This approach can increase access[1] to care, especially for individuals in remote or underserved areas, reduce costs, and provide convenient and efficient management of various health conditions.[2] A 2022 survey[3] by the American Medical Association found that 60% of participating physicians agreed or strongly agreed that telehealth facilitated their delivery of high-quality care. Additionally, over 80% of respondents indicated that telehealth improved patient access to care.

Historical Context and Evolution

The invention of telemedicine cannot be attributed to a single entity or organization. Telemedicine, using telecommunication and information technology to provide healthcare from a distance, has evolved through contributions from various sectors, institutions, and individuals.

Telemedicine has its roots in early telecommunications and radio technologies.

The history of telemedicine is a fascinating chronicle of innovation, adaptation, and the relentless pursuit of extending healthcare's reach through technology. It's a story that parallels the evolution of communication technologies, reflecting society's broader technological advances and its ever-changing healthcare needs.

Early Foundations (1860s–1950s)

The seeds of telemedicine were planted with the advent of mid-19th-century communication technology. One of the first instances of telemedicine was in the 1860s, during the American Civil War when the telegraph was used to inform medical teams about injured soldiers.[4] Then, in 1906, Willem Einthoven, the inventor of the electrocardiograph, transmitted electrocardiograms (ECGs) over telephone lines.[5] This groundbreaking work later earned Einthoven a Nobel Prize and laid the conceptual foundation for remote medical diagnosis.

By the 1920s, another pioneering development occurred with ship-to-shore radio communications.[6] Ships at sea, isolated from immediate medical care, would use radio to seek medical advice from clinicians on land — a lifeline for distressed sailors and a primitive form of telemedicine.

With every new telecommunication technology, it seemed a new type of telemedicine was innovated. After the invention of the television, for example, surgeons at the Johns Hopkins Hospital used television to educate surgeons. In 1944, Hopkin's surgeons broadcasted an operation using a closed-circuit television to many surgeons.[7]

Initial Experiments (1960s–1970s)

Murphy and Bird first proposed the phrase "telemedicine" in an article in the *American Journal of Public Health* in 1974. They described how physicians at the emergency ward at the Massachusetts General Hospital provided medical care to over 1,000 patients at the medical station of the Logan International Airport using a two-way audiovisual microwave circuit.

Telemedicine's potential took a significant leap forward with the involvement of the U.S. space program. NASA's concern for astronaut health in space led to the development of biomedical telemetry — transmitting biometric data back to Earth[8] during the Project Mercury missions. To continuously evaluate the astronauts' health and to provide immediate medical advice, teams of medical monitors were positioned at 18 sites across the globe.[9] This demonstrated that by using telecommunications, physicians could have greater availability and provide care beyond what was thought possible.

These technologies would soon find their way into terrestrial applications, most notably through the Space Technology Applied to Rural Papago Advanced Health Care (STARPAHC) program. The STARPAHC program was an innovative project developed in the 1970s that represented one of the earliest uses of telemedicine.[10] This project was a joint venture between NASA and the U.S. Public Health Service to explore the potential of space technology in improving healthcare delivery to remote locations.

The primary goal of the STARPAHC program was to provide healthcare services to the Papago Indian Reservation in Arizona, a region with limited access to medical facilities. The project used telecommunication technology to connect patients in this remote area with physicians and nearby medical facilities. It involved transmitting medical data, such as X-rays and ECGs, and even facilitated interactive consultations via video.

The STARPAHC program demonstrated that telemedicine could effectively extend healthcare's reach, particularly to underserved populations in isolated areas. It was an essential precursor to today's telehealth systems, showing that space technology could have practical applications on Earth, especially in medical care and public health. The project served as a proof of concept for telemedicine and laid the groundwork for its future development and expansion.

Around the same time, Wittson and Dutton[11] at the University of Nebraska started using interactive telemedicine via a bidirectional closed-circuit television in psychiatry to provide medical education and training. Later, they used this technology to conduct group therapy sessions "at a distance."[12]

Technological Advancements (1980s–1990s)

The proliferation of cable television networks and the nascent internet in the 1980s and 1990s facilitated a broader adoption of telemedicine. During this era, the term "telemedicine" began to be widely recognized. One example was the use of teleconferencing by radiologists, which allowed for sharing of patient images and collaborative diagnoses across distances, revolutionizing radiology.

This period also saw the development of more structured regulatory frameworks to govern the use of telemedicine. The American Telemedicine Association (ATA), founded in 1993, began to establish guidelines and standards for telemedicine practices.[13]

Even the U.S. military helped advance this technology. The U.S. military's interest in telemedicine has primarily been driven by the need to provide medical care to service members stationed in remote and combat areas.[14] By the 1990s, the U.S. military had begun to invest more significantly in telemedicine, using it during various military operations to provide care and conduct medical consultations for troops deployed overseas. The U.S. Army's first usage of video-enabled care was in 1993 in Somalia, followed by expansion during the 1994–1995 Balkan conflicts.[15]

The U.S. Army has continued to develop and use telemedicine solutions, primarily through the Telemedicine & Advanced Technology Research Center (TATRC), headquartered at Fort Detrick in Frederick, Maryland.[16] The TATRC has been at the forefront of researching and deploying new healthcare technologies for military medicine and the broader medical community.

Mainstream Adoption (2000s–2010s)

The turn of the century heralded the era of broadband and the ubiquity of the internet, significantly improving telemedicine services' quality and reliability. Video conferencing became smoother and more secure, allowing for real-time interactions between patients and healthcare providers.

Mobile health, or mHealth, emerged with the smartphone revolution, exemplified by the launch of Apple's iPhone in 2007. The Global Observatory for eHealth of the World Health Organization defines mHealth as "medical and public health practice supported by mobile devices, such as mobile phones, patient monitoring devices, personal digital assistants, and other wireless devices."[17] As mobile telecommunication technology improved, health applications became commonplace, allowing patients to track their health metrics and consult with physicians from anywhere. These are reasonable solutions and tools to collect and provide information on patient health and vital status to medical providers. One of the benefits of mHealth is that it can enhance the continuity of care through better maintenance of patient medical records.[18] Direct and indirect patient costs can be reduced by lowering the frequency of clinic visits and[19] hospitalizations.[20,21]

The Veterans Health Administration adopted a wide array of telehealth services, demonstrating how extensive a telemedicine program could be.[22]

Electronic health records (EHRs) systems, becoming the standard in healthcare, incorporated telemedicine features, creating a seamless digital environment for remote healthcare delivery.[23]

Maturation and Expansion (2020s)

The 2020s, while still in their infancy, have already been defined by the global COVID-19 pandemic, which thrust telemedicine into the spotlight like never before. Social distancing measures necessitated the rapid adoption of telemedicine as a critical tool in healthcare delivery. Policies and regulations were quickly adapted to facilitate this, with the U.S. government expanding the Medicare coverage for telemedicine services.

The pandemic also sparked global interest in telemedicine to address healthcare disparities. For example, in India, the eSanjeevani initiative has provided millions of online consultations, showcasing the potential for telemedicine in resource-limited settings.

In 2020, a study on the U.S. telemedicine market stated that more than 75% of U.S. hospitals had some form of telemedicine program.

A study published in *JAMA Internal Medicine* reported that telehealth visits increased nearly 40-fold from prepandemic levels and comprised nearly half of all Medicare visits at the pandemic's peak.

A report by McKinsey stated that the demand for telehealth exploded during the pandemic, estimating that physicians saw between 50 and 175 times more patients via telehealth than they did before the outbreak.[24]

Another article published in *Mortality and Morbidity Weekly Report*[25] stated that between January and March 2020, most encounters were from patients seeking care for conditions other than COVID-19.

Additionally, a position paper[26] from the COVID-19 pandemic highlighted the acceleration of telemedicine adoption globally. The paper discussed the status or maturity of telemedicine implementation across various regions and the developments or changes adopted during COVID-19. For instance, in countries like Singapore and India, significant government efforts were to support telemedicine services and incorporate them into the existing healthcare framework.

Telemedicine's history is a testament to technological progress and a narrative of healthcare's adaptability. It has bridged distances, connected disparate communities to care, and shown resilience in the face of global challenges. As we look into the future, the continued evolution of telemedicine promises to transform healthcare delivery further, making it more accessible, efficient, and patient-centered than ever before.

Regulatory Changes that Facilitated Telemedicine

Several regulatory changes have facilitated the adoption of telemedicine in the United States, particularly in response to evolving healthcare needs and technological advancements:

The Ryan Haight Act Amendment

The Ryan Haight Online Pharmacy Consumer Protection Act of 2008 was initially a barrier to telemedicine because it required a face-to-face examination before prescribing controlled substances. However, with the rise of telemedicine, there were calls to amend this act to allow for prescriptions via telemedicine under specific circumstances. Therefore, the Ryan Haight Act Amendment[27] was passed on March 27, 2020, to ease regulations on prescribing medications via telemedicine during the COVID-19 public health emergency. This amendment suspends the Ryan Haight Act's requirement for a prior patient evaluation before prescribing controlled substances through telemedicine. It permits healthcare providers to prescribe certain controlled substances through telemedicine without an initial face-to-face patient encounter, enabling greater use of telemedicine to continue treating chronic conditions remotely.

This amendment allowed more flexibility for telemedicine prescribing throughout the COVID-19 pandemic, as regular visits to maintain prescriptions for conditions such as chronic pain faced obstacles with physical distancing policies.

Reimbursement Policies

Historically, reimbursement for telemedicine services was limited, which was a significant barrier to its adoption. Changes in Medicare reimbursement policies have gradually expanded coverage for telemedicine services. These changes include the following:

The Medicare Telehealth Parity Act of 2014 proposed to expand the scope of telehealth services covered by Medicare.

The 21st Century Cures Act,[28] passed in 2016, aimed to promote the use of telehealth in various ways, including encouraging its use within Medicare and Medicaid. The Act proposed a phased approach to expand Medicare reimbursement for telehealth services. It aimed to modernize the payment system and extend telehealth coverage to all federally qualified health centers, rural health clinics, and homes.[29] This act is intended to broaden the scope of telehealth services beyond rural areas to include urban areas and to cover various healthcare providers and services, including remote patient monitoring and asynchronous telehealth services. It was an effort to bring Medicare payment policies up to date with technological capabilities and healthcare delivery trends.

The CONNECT for Health Act[30]

The Creating Opportunities Now for Necessary and Effective Care Technologies (CONNECT) for Health Act is a bipartisan bill proposed in

2019 to further expand Medicare coverage for telemedicine services and remove some of the geographic and setting limitations that were previously in place. This act aimed to build on temporary telehealth policies instituted during the COVID-19 public health emergency by permanently eliminating restrictions on eligible telehealth practitioners, authorizing the Centers for Medicare & Medicaid Services (CMS) to reimburse for more telehealth services, and allowing telehealth services regardless of geographic locations. The CONNECT for Health Act intended to increase telehealth access for Medicare beneficiaries to improve health outcomes by enabling more convenient care from home. The passage of this act was projected to rapidly accelerate telemedicine adoption by providing consistent reimbursement policies that incentivize providers to deliver virtual care. The bill also calls for a study on telehealth use during the pandemic to guide future policies.

Public Health Emergency Waivers

During the COVID-19 public health emergency, the CMS issued an unprecedented 1135 telehealth waiver granting provisional emergency telehealth policy changes to mitigate the pandemic.[31] The "1135 waiver" refers to section 1135 of the Social Security Act, which authorizes the Secretary of the U.S. Department of Health and Human Services (HHS) to temporarily waive or modify certain Medicare, Medicaid, and CHIP requirements during declared emergencies to ensure sufficient healthcare items and services are available.

These waivers provided extensive temporary regulatory flexibility to accelerate the rapid adoption of telemedicine services and reimbursement. Fundamental changes enabled under the 1135 waiver included eliminating originating site restrictions and geographic limits, covering audio-only visits, allowing interstate practice, and reimbursing telehealth services at the same rates as in-person care. This waiver allowed Medicare to pay for an office, hospital, and other visits furnished via telehealth nationwide, including in patients' homes.

A report examining CMS claims data found that 10.1 million telehealth visits were made for Medicare fee-for-service beneficiaries in just 28 days after the waiver, drastically increasing access in a highly condensed period.

It is expanding the types of healthcare providers who can offer tele-health services.[32]

Among the significant temporary telehealth policy changes instituted by the CMS during the COVID-19 pandemic was the significantly expanding practitioner eligibility to provide and bill for telehealth services. Prior restrictive policies only allowed physicians and certain practitioners to deliver and be reimbursed for telehealth. However, emergency policies enabled hospitals, home health agencies, hospices, outpatient rehabilitation facilities, critical access hospitals, rural health clinics, and federally qualified health centers to furnish broader virtual care services. Enabling additional healthcare providers and facility types to offer telemedicine helped rapidly expand access and capacity, meeting the surging health needs. Over 100 temporary coding and coverage policies were implemented just for Medicare services to reimburse more practitioners delivering telehealth across the continuum of care. Broadening telehealth eligibility helped mobilize more comprehensive health system capacity through telemedicine when confronting the pandemic's extraordinary demands on care delivery.

Health Insurance Portability and Accountability Act Enforcement Discretion

To further facilitate the rapid expansion of telehealth access amid the challenges of the COVID-19 pandemic, the HHS announced notification of enforcement discretion for the Health Insurance Portability and Accountability Act (HIPAA) privacy regulations in March 2020.[33] This allowed medical providers additional flexibility to provide telehealth services through everyday communication technologies, including Apple FaceTime, Facebook Messenger, Google Hangouts, Zoom, and Skype. Healthcare providers were permitted to use these popular non-public-facing video chat platforms to offer telehealth to patients despite such platforms typically needing to fully comply with the HIPAA rules. Temporary relaxation of restrictions enabled more widespread telemedicine adoption to reduce barriers during unprecedented demands on health systems. This HIPAA enforcement discretion expired on May 11 2023, when the public health emergency ended.[34]

Licensure Flexibility

State-based licensure requirements have been a significant barrier to telemedicine. Many states have started participating in the Interstate Medical Licensure Compact, which offers a streamlined process for physicians to become licensed in multiple states, facilitating telemedicine across state lines.

Cross-State Practice

During the COVID-19 pandemic, many states temporarily allowed out-of-state healthcare providers to treat their residents via telehealth without obtaining additional state licenses, recognizing the importance of telemedicine in the pandemic response.

These regulatory changes, among others, have played a crucial role in increasing telemedicine adoption by removing previous barriers, increasing access to services, and ensuring providers can receive adequate reimbursement for telehealth services.

Bridging Healthcare Gaps

The role of internet availability and the digital divide is critical in determining the accessibility and effectiveness of telemedicine services. Telemedicine's potential to bridge healthcare gaps, especially in rural and underserved urban settings, heavily depends on reliable, high-speed internet access. With it, the benefits of telemedicine can be fully realized.

The Role of Internet Availability

Internet availability is the backbone of telemedicine services.[35] High-speed broadband enables video conferencing, real-time data transfer of medical records, and remote monitoring of patients' health. In urban areas, where high-speed internet is more widely available, telemedicine can seamlessly integrate into healthcare delivery systems, providing convenience and improving efficiency.

However, limited internet availability can be a significant barrier in rural areas. According to the Federal Communications Commission (FCC), as of 2021, approximately 22.3% of rural Americans lack access to high-speed internet, compared to just 1.5% of urban Americans.[36,37] This disparity in access creates a digital divide that can hinder the reach of telemedicine services.

Impact of the Digital Divide on Telemedicine Access

The digital divide refers to the gap between demographics and regions with reliable access to modern information and communication technologies and those without it. This divide creates disparities in healthcare access, particularly in telemedicine, as it disproportionately affects older adults, low-income families, and certain racial and ethnic groups. For instance, a Pew Research Center study found that 29% of adults aged 65 and older lack home broadband, limiting their ability to participate in virtual consultations or use online patient portals.[38]

Without reliable internet, affected populations may face significant barriers to telehealth services such as scheduling appointments, consulting with specialists, or accessing electronic health records (EHRs). Beyond access, digital literacy — the ability to use technology effectively — further compounds the issue, especially among older adults and underserved communities. The result is not only delayed care but also poorer health outcomes due to limited opportunities for timely interventions, chronic disease management, and preventive care.

Efforts to bridge the digital divide are crucial for reducing these disparities. Programs such as the Federal Communications Commission's (FCC) Affordable Connectivity Program provide subsidies for internet access to low-income households. Community initiatives, such as digital literacy workshops, are also helping individuals develop the skills needed to navigate telehealth platforms. By addressing both access and literacy, healthcare systems can ensure telemedicine benefits reach all populations, fostering more equitable health outcomes.

Telemedicine's Reach and Impact on Patient Outcomes

The impact of telemedicine on patient outcomes can be profound, particularly when it increases access to healthcare services. Studies have shown that telemedicine can lead to the following:

- Improved access to primary and specialty care, especially for patients in rural areas who are far from healthcare providers.
- Enhanced chronic disease management through regular monitoring and patient engagement.
- Reduced travel time and costs associated with accessing healthcare services.
- Decreased emergency room visits and hospital readmissions due to better outpatient management and follow-up care.
- The federal government has labeled 80% of rural U.S. communities — in which 20% of all Americans live — as medically underserved.[39] In rural settings, where the distance to healthcare facilities can be a significant barrier, telemedicine has been shown to improve patient outcomes by providing timely access to care. For instance, a study published in the *Journal of the American Medical Association* (*JAMA*) found that telemedicine interventions in rural areas improved outcomes for patients with chronic conditions, such as diabetes and heart disease.[40]
- Conversely, in urban settings, where the density of healthcare resources is higher, the impact of telemedicine may be more focused on improving the efficiency of healthcare delivery and reducing wait times for appointments. Yet, even in these settings, the digital divide can impact marginalized communities, underlining the need for inclusive policies and investment in digital infrastructure to ensure equitable access to telemedicine services for all populations.

Addressing the digital divide is therefore not only a matter of technological infrastructure but also one of health equity. Policymakers, healthcare providers, and community leaders must work together to ensure that the benefits of telemedicine reach all segments of the population, regardless of geographical location or socioeconomic status.

Best Practices for Telemedicine Appointments and Follow-Up

For telemedicine to realize its full potential, the proficiency of healthcare professionals in navigating virtual appointments is essential.[41] The best practices for telemedicine appointments and follow-ups encompass not only the utilization of technology but also the skillful interaction with patients in a virtual space. Here's how training and standardization can be addressed to enhance the quality of telemedicine.

Training Healthcare Professionals for Telemedicine

Understanding Telemedicine Platforms: Imagine a scenario where a physician logs into a telemedicine session and spends the first 10 minutes troubleshooting audio issues. To avoid this, comprehensive training on the technical use of telemedicine platforms is vital.[41] Providers should be adept at troubleshooting common technical problems to minimize disruptions during patient consultations.

Clinical Skills in a Virtual Environment[42]

Consider a dermatologist assessing a skin lesion over video. Training should prepare providers to guide patients in angling the camera or choosing lighting that allows for the best visual assessment possible, compensating for the inability to physically examine the patient. The COVID-19 pandemic necessitated a rapid shift to providing healthcare through virtual and telemedicine platforms. Healthcare professionals have had to quickly adapt and develop new clinical skills tailored for telehealth environments rather than traditional in-person care. As the cited source discusses, effectively assessing patients, building rapport, and conducting exams pose new challenges in a video encounter. Clinicians need training to hone telemedicine-specific approaches to gather clinical information, perceive nonverbal cues virtually, and decide on interventions while unable to physically examine the patient. The pandemic revealed widescale telehealth implementation is likely inevitable, so purposefully fostering relevant telemedicine skills prepares providers to deliver quality, patient-centered care regardless of the setting. Updating clinical education and training for virtual care settings ensures healthcare professionals can safely and sensitively translate in-person expertise to telehealth delivery.

Communication and Etiquette

Effective communication in telemedicine encompasses much more than verbal discussion alone.

As nonverbal cues comprise a primary conduit for conveying emotion and nurturing rapport, mastering visualization techniques is essential for impactful video visits. However, through a screen, clinicians can overlook 50% or more of the subtle body language dynamics evident in person.[43] Providers should refine skills by picking up on visual signals such as microexpressions or postural shifts indicative of discomfort. Techniques such as sitting sufficiently distanced to monitor gestural signs of pain, frequently meeting eyes to perceive reactions, and verbal checks on mood state facilitate richer assessment. Since appropriate eye contact varies cross-culturally, customizing to each patient's comfort allows a more meaningful connection. In essence, by honing visual acuity and verbal diligence for subtle virtual interactions, providers enhance telemedicine delivery, avoid communication gaps that impair outcomes, and better emulate the patient-centeredness of in-person care.

Providers need to be proficient in deciphering visual cues and subtle body language during video consultations, as these nonverbal signals convey vital information. Through a screen, signs of patient discomfort, uncertainty, or disengagement may manifest more delicately than during in-person examinations. A clinician's attentiveness to narrowing eyes, frequent shifting, strained expressions, and fleeting microexpressions allows them to preemptively address unspoken concerns. These ongoing assessments of mood and disposition require particular focus in video encounters.

Specific telemedicine etiquette can aid engagement with these nuanced virtual atmospherics. Adopting proper posture, limiting distracting gestures, and maintaining culturally appropriate eye contact emulate in-person inclusivity. Brief verbal check-ins on comfort also help providers validate patients' potential worries in an unfamiliar process. While mastering verbal guidance remains imperative, aptitude in perceiving visual emotional states and refined video visit conduct uphold patient-centered telemedicine delivery. This multifaceted communication competence engenders trust and assurance essential for optimal telehealth outcomes. In essence, by honing sensory and interpersonal techniques tailored for telemedicine's unique human dynamics, clinicians facilitate impactful virtual care on par with gold-standard in-office standards.

Legal and Ethical Competence[44]

As telehealth technologies rapidly transform healthcare delivery, healthcare providers must prioritize legal and ethical competence to ensure safe, effective, and patient-centered care.[45]

Understanding and adhering to legal frameworks surrounding licensure, data security, patient consent, and reimbursement is imperative.[46] This requires ongoing education and staying abreast of evolving regulations across various jurisdictions.

However, legal compliance alone is insufficient. Ethical considerations demand attention as well. Building strong therapeutic relationships remotely requires adapting communication skills and utilizing technology effectively. Providers must prioritize accessibility and ensure an equitable access to telehealth services regardless of patients' backgrounds or technological capabilities.

Furthermore, understanding the limitations of telehealth is critical. Recognizing situations where in-person care is necessary and upholding professional boundaries are essential aspects of ethical telehealth practice. This includes avoiding conflicts of interest, particularly regarding remote prescriptions of controlled substances.

Developing legal and ethical competence requires proactive engagement from healthcare providers. Participating in specialized training programs, utilizing online resources, seeking mentorship from experienced practitioners, and collaborating with legal and ethics experts are valuable pathways to achieving this crucial skill set.

By prioritizing legal and ethical considerations, healthcare professionals can ensure that telehealth services are delivered in a responsible and patient-centered manner.[47] This fosters trust in this transformative field and empowers telehealth to reach its full potential in improving global healthcare delivery.

Cultural Competence[48]

According to the 2020 U.S. Census, racial and ethnic minorities make up about a third of the U.S. population.[49] Therefore, telehealth training must prioritize cultural competency to ensure providers can adeptly serve diverse populations. Certain communities may have differing attitudes, norms, or barriers regarding technology-facilitated care. Clinicians require guidance accounting for how factors such as health beliefs, communication styles, or privacy perceptions influence virtual visit effectiveness across cultures. For instance, some racial groups exhibit lower telehealth uptake, partly attributable to a lack of digital literacy or linguistic fluency, impeding engagement. Age and income disparities in technology access also disproportionately impact adoption. Formally addressing such variability allows more patient-centered and ethical practice. Tailoring communication approaches to be inclusive of cultural variances can also build essential trust and rapport. Techniques such as proactively leveraging interpreter services or pointedly discussing any uncertainties about telemedicine procedures promote personalized support.

Standardization across Healthcare Systems

A cornerstone for successful telehealth standardization across healthcare systems is essential to optimize the adoption and impact of telehealth technologies. Interoperability—the ability of diverse systems and organizations to exchange and use health information seamlessly—depends on unified frameworks and consistent standards. Without standardization, telemedicine tools are often developed in silos, resulting in fragmented virtual care infrastructures that hinder the efficient exchange of data. This fragmentation poses significant challenges for patients transitioning between providers and for clinicians attempting to deliver cohesive, high-quality care. The following are some important areas of standardization:

Key Data Standards

Fast Healthcare Interoperability Resources (FHIR)

FHIR is a framework that uses modern web technologies and application programming interfaces (APIs) to enable the secure exchange of health information. It allows developers to build applications that access EHR data across different systems seamlessly.

Systematized Nomenclature of Medicine (SNOMED)

SNOMED is a standardized medical terminology system that ensures uniform documentation of clinical information, reducing inconsistencies in patient records.

RxNorm

RxNorm provides standardized naming conventions for medications, facilitating accurate prescription management and reducing medication errors.

United States Core Data for Interoperability (USCDI)

USCDI defines a minimum set of standardized health data elements required for nationwide exchange, including demographics, clinical notes, and laboratory results.

Together, these standards address the technical and semantic challenges of interoperability, paving the way for more effective telehealth delivery.

Progress and Persistent Challenges

Over the past decade, the adoption of these standards has advanced interoperability in healthcare. For example, FHIR APIs have enabled third-party applications to integrate seamlessly with EHR systems, allowing patients to access their medical records and share data with providers effortlessly. Similarly, SNOMED and RxNorm have standardized clinical terminology and medication documentation, reducing errors and improving continuity of care.

Despite these advancements, universal interoperability remains elusive. Barriers include incomplete access to patient records, inconsistent implementation of standards across healthcare organizations, and limited two-way data exchange between differing EHR systems. Device integration protocols, such as those enabling remote monitoring devices to communicate with EHRs, also require further standardization to ensure seamless data flow.

The Role of Standardization in Telehealth

Standardization benefits not only the technical side of healthcare but also the patient and provider experience:

- **For Patients:** Unified standards simplify navigation of telehealth platforms, reducing confusion when accessing virtual care. For example, a patient using a mobile app built on FHIR standards can seamlessly share their health data with specialists at different facilities.
- **For Providers:** Consistent standards ensure that clinicians receive complete, accurate patient information, enabling them to offer personalized care. Training programs based on these standards empower providers to deliver exceptional virtual care, regardless of their facility's specific EHR system.

Moreover, widespread standardization enables the establishment of quality and accountability metrics.

By benchmarking outcomes across systems, healthcare organizations can identify best practices, improve telehealth delivery, and enhance patient outcomes.

Looking Ahead: The Path to Widespread Interoperability

To fully realize the promise of telehealth, healthcare systems must prioritize standardization:

- **Device Integration:** Adopting protocols that allow wearables and remote monitoring devices to share data with EHRs will enhance coordinated care.
- **Collaboration:** Partnerships between healthcare organizations, technology vendors, and standardization bodies like HL7 are critical for ensuring widespread adoption.
- **Policy Support:** Initiatives like the Office of the National Coordinator for Health Information Technology's (ONC) mandate for FHIR-based APIs highlight the importance of governmental involvement in promoting interoperability.

By embracing unified standards, healthcare systems can overcome technical and logistical barriers, ensuring that telehealth technologies work cohesively to improve accessibility and patient outcomes.

Creating Universal Protocols

The establishment of universal protocols for telehealth is essential to ensuring consistent and high-quality care. Healthcare professionals must navigate various telehealth technologies; standard protocols provide a framework for delivering services effectively and safely. These protocols encompass patient privacy, clinical workflows, and technical standards. They foster a uniform patient experience and streamline care coordination, which is critical given the diverse telehealth platforms in use. For example, developing a standardized checklist for pre-appointment setup can ensure that all providers across a healthcare system are prepared for telemedicine visits.[50] This might include steps for secure login, environment setup, and patient identity verification.[51]

Accreditation and Certification in Telehealth

As telehealth becomes an integral part of healthcare delivery, ensuring quality and competency in this rapidly evolving field is paramount. Accreditation and certification programs play a critical role in building trust among patients, providers, and stakeholders. These programs establish standards for telehealth practice, evaluate providers' adherence to those standards, and recognize those who meet the highest benchmarks of excellence. Several key organizations lead the way in telehealth accreditation and certification:

- **Utilization Review Accreditation Commission (URAC):** URAC is an independent nonprofit organization known for setting high-quality standards in healthcare. Its telehealth accreditation program evaluates the operational efficiency, patient safety, and clinical quality of telehealth providers. URAC's emphasis on innovation ensures that telehealth practices remain adaptable to emerging technologies and challenges.
- **American Telemedicine Association (ATA):** As one of the earliest advocates for telehealth, the ATA develops comprehensive guidelines and best practices for virtual care. Its accreditation programs focus on ensuring that telehealth services meet rigorous clinical and operational standards, fostering trust and reliability in the industry.
- **Accreditation Commission for Health Care (ACHC):** ACHC provides accreditation services tailored to telehealth providers, with a focus on enhancing organizational efficiency and improving patient outcomes. By setting clear benchmarks, ACHC helps providers deliver consistent, high-quality virtual care.

These organizations ensure that telehealth providers demonstrate the knowledge, skills, and competencies needed to meet the demands of modern virtual care. For instance, telemedicine certification programs for nurses set critical benchmarks for their role in facilitating virtual consultations, triaging patients, and managing care plans. Certified nurses ensure that patients receive safe, effective, and empathetic care, regardless of whether they are seen in person or online.

The Importance of Accreditation

Accreditation programs are essential for several reasons:

- **For Patients:** Accreditation provides assurance that telehealth services adhere to high-quality standards, improving patient confidence and satisfaction. Accredited programs often emphasize patient safety, data privacy, and ease of access.
- **For Providers:** Certification programs establish clear benchmarks for telehealth competencies, empowering providers to deliver exceptional care. These programs also foster professional growth by keeping providers informed about the latest best practices in telehealth.
- **For Healthcare Organizations:** Accreditation ensures operational consistency and regulatory compliance, reducing risks and enhancing efficiency. It also facilitates benchmarking, enabling organizations to compare outcomes and identify areas for improvement.

Examples of Accreditation's Impact

Consider a hospital implementing telehealth services to reach rural communities. Accreditation by URAC or ACHC ensures that the hospital's telehealth program uses secure communication platforms, adheres to privacy regulations, and maintains clinical quality. Patients in remote areas benefit from reliable access to specialists, while providers gain the tools to deliver care with confidence.

Similarly, ATA guidelines help clinics design virtual care programs that integrate seamlessly with existing workflows. By aligning with these guidelines, clinics can avoid pitfalls such as fragmented data systems or inconsistent care protocols, ultimately improving patient outcomes.

Building a Global Perspective

Accreditation is not only vital in the United States but also in the global telehealth landscape. In countries with rapidly expanding telemedicine programs, adopting international standards like those from ATA or URAC ensures quality and consistency across borders. This global approach fosters collaboration and improves access to high-quality virtual care worldwide.

Conclusion

Accreditation and certification are the backbone of high-quality telehealth services. Organizations such as URAC, ATA, and ACHC provide the frameworks needed to ensure that telehealth providers meet the highest standards of care. By embracing these programs, patients can trust the care they receive, providers can deliver services with confidence, and healthcare organizations can operate more effectively. As telehealth continues to transform healthcare delivery, accreditation will remain a key driver of innovation, trust, and excellence.

Continuous Professional Development

Just as cardiologists stay abreast of the latest in heart health, so too must telemedicine practitioners remain current with technological and methodological advancements. Regular training modules or e-learning programs can support this continuous education. The Association of American Medical Colleges (AAMC) has outlined telehealth competencies[52] that serve as a guide for the educational and professional development of physicians at various stages of their careers. These competencies span several domains, including patient safety, access and equity, communication, data collection, technology use, and legal and ethical practices in telehealth.

Quality Assurance and Feedback Mechanisms

The essential nature of telehealth as a delivery platform for healthcare services, rather than a distinct type of care, necessitates its adherence to the same standards and quality metrics as in-person care, wherever feasible and appropriate.[53] When the unique characteristics of telehealth dictate a need for adjustment, such adjustments should be made to existing measures, not involve complete reinvention. Furthermore, when supported by evidence and established standards of care, measure stewards should strive to maintain consistency in standards and anticipated outcomes for services delivered via telehealth.

Effective quality assurance (QA) frameworks encompass comprehensive assessments of telehealth infrastructure, clinical processes, and patient outcomes while incorporating feedback from patients, providers, and other stakeholders. The goals of an effective QA framework include enhanced patient and provider experiences, a commitment to health equity, consistent monitoring of technical performance and uptime, responsible financial management, and positive clinical outcomes.[54]

This feedback plays a vital role in identifying areas for improvement, adapting services to address evolving needs, and fostering a culture of continuous quality improvement within telehealth programs.

To ensure effectiveness, QA and feedback mechanisms should be integrated into the telehealth program design and implemented throughout its lifecycle. This includes regular audits and performance monitoring, standardized patient experience surveys, and open communication channels for patient feedback and concerns. By systematically collecting and analyzing feedback, telehealth providers can identify and address issues related to access, affordability, patient–provider communication, and technology usability. This data-driven approach to QA and feedback allows for proactive adjustments to improve service delivery and enhance patient satisfaction.

An example here would be implementing a standardized patient survey following telehealth appointments, which would provide direct feedback on the patient experience and highlight areas for provider improvement.

Interdisciplinary Collaboration

Telemedicine often requires several different types of healthcare providers to work together to care for a patient. Healthcare professionals seeking to function within interdisciplinary teams must embrace collaboration, actively engage in continuous learning and development opportunities, and prioritize transparent communication.[55] Building a cohesive team requires meticulous coordination, collaborative effort, and a culture of openness. Encourage, for instance, a virtual tumor board where specialists from different locations come together via telehealth platforms to discuss complex cancer cases, combining diverse expertise to improve patient outcomes.

With targeted training and standardization, healthcare providers can conduct telemedicine visits that are not only efficient but also empathetic, bridging the physical distance to deliver care that is as close to in-person quality as possible.

Privacy and Security in Telemedicine

In the digital age, privacy and security are at the forefront of healthcare conversations, particularly regarding telemedicine. Telemedicine's ability to transcend geographic barriers brings forth unique challenges in safeguarding patient information. Indeed, telehealth will not succeed if privacy and security risks are not addressed.[56]

In a systematic review by Houser et al.,[57] three critical risk factors contributing to privacy and security concerns in telehealth were identified: environmental (limited private space for vulnerable populations and difficulties in sharing sensitive information remotely), technological (data security vulnerabilities, limited internet, and technology availability), and operational (reimbursement uncertainties, payer denials, technology accessibility challenges, and insufficient training and educational resources). These findings provide valuable insights for governments, policymakers, and healthcare organizations to develop robust telehealth privacy and security strategies.

The following section explores the intricacies of privacy and security in telemedicine, highlighting why they are critical and how healthcare providers can address these concerns.

The Importance of Privacy and Security in Telemedicine

Telemedicine inherently involves the exchange of sensitive health information over communication networks. This exchange increases the risk of unauthorized access, data breaches, and potential privacy violations. The

HIPAA sets the standard for protecting sensitive patient data in the United States. However, the expansion of telemedicine services raises questions about the adequacy of existing privacy and security measures.

Data Transmission Security

Data transmitted during telemedicine sessions must be encrypted to prevent interception by unauthorized parties. However, the use of various platforms, some of which may not be designed for healthcare purposes, can lead to vulnerabilities where data are exposed.

Device and Endpoint Security

Telemedicine often involves the use of personal devices by both providers and patients. These devices can be susceptible to malware and other security threats, which can compromise the confidentiality and integrity of health information.

Authentication and Access Controls

Ensuring that only authorized individuals have access to telemedicine platforms and patient data is essential. Weak authentication processes can lead to unauthorized access, putting patient information at risk.

Best Practices for Ensuring Privacy and Security

Adherence to Regulatory Standards: Healthcare providers must ensure that their telemedicine practices comply with HIPAA regulations and other relevant standards, which may involve using HIPAA-compliant telemedicine platforms and secure messaging services.

Regular Security Audits

Conducting regular security audits can help identify potential vulnerabilities within telemedicine systems. For example, a clinic might hire a third-party cybersecurity firm to test their systems' defenses periodically.

Staff Training

Educating healthcare staff about the importance of security practices is crucial. Regular training sessions can help staff recognize phishing attempts, understand the importance of strong passwords, and stay updated on best practices for digital hygiene.

Patient Education

Patients also play a role in maintaining their privacy and should be educated about how to secure their devices and internet connections. A simple step such as instructing patients to use private Wi-Fi networks rather than public ones during telehealth sessions can significantly reduce risk.

Use of Secure Platforms and Tools

Healthcare providers should use telemedicine platforms that offer end-to-end encryption, secure data storage, and robust user authentication protocols.[58] For instance, a telemedicine platform may implement two-factor authentication to ensure that the person logging in is indeed the patient or the provider.

Incident Response Planning

In the event of a security breach, having an incident response plan in place ensures that providers can act swiftly to mitigate harm. This plan might include immediate steps to secure data, assess the extent of a breach, and notify affected patients.

Ethical Considerations

Telemedicine, heralded as a beacon of innovation in healthcare, offers a myriad of advantages such as convenience, cost-effectiveness, and the ability to transcend geographical barriers. However, its rapid growth brings to light several ethical implications that warrant careful consideration. Among these are the imperatives to ensure equitable access and to avoid potential disruptions to the continuity of care. This section explores these ethical dimensions and the importance of addressing them within the telemedicine framework.

Equitable Access to Telemedicine

The promise of telemedicine lies in its potential to democratize healthcare, making medical consultations and health monitoring available to all, regardless of the location. Yet, this promise remains unfulfilled for many. A comprehensive telemedicine system encompasses various entities, stakeholders, providers, and patients across diverse specialties or conditions. This complex ecosystem, with its inherent diversity, can harbor conflicting practices, cultures, regulations, and communication styles, making the implementation of telemedicine a multifaceted and challenging undertaking.[59] An example of this complexity is the digital divide. The digital divide — a term that encapsulates the discrepancies in access to information and communication technologies — presents a significant ethical challenge.[60] Those patients without reliable internet access, particularly in rural areas or among disadvantaged communities, may find themselves excluded from telemedicine's benefits.

Moreover, there are disparities in digital literacy. A recent study by Drake et al.[61] revealed that African American and male patients were less likely to utilize telemedicine (both phone and video) compared to white and female patients. Additionally, within the telemedicine group, African American, publicly insured, and older patients were less likely to use video consultations compared to white, commercially insured, and younger patients. For deaf and non-English speaking patients, effective communication is particularly difficult; the use of skilled medical interpreters is essential to provide fair virtual treatment.

The elderly and some socioeconomically disadvantaged groups may struggle with the technical skills required to engage in telemedicine effectively. While many patients are interested in video visits, they are interested in low-tech solutions and at-the-elbow support to feel confident in using the technology. An ethical telemedicine practice must, therefore, not only ensure the availability of technology but also provide the necessary support and education to enable all patients to use these services effectively.

Care Continuity in Telemedicine

Another ethical consideration is the continuity of care. Telemedicine can either enhance or disrupt the traditional patient–provider relationship. On one hand, telemedicine can facilitate ongoing health management, especially for chronic conditions, through regular virtual checkups and monitoring.[62] On the other hand, there's a risk of fragmented[63] care when patients use telemedicine services that do not coordinate with their primary care providers or when they opt for on-demand care from providers who are not familiar with their medical history.

To maintain continuity of care, telemedicine services must be integrated into the broader healthcare system. This involves careful record-keeping and communication between telemedicine providers and patients' primary care doctors. Additionally, ethical telemedicine practice should prioritize the establishment of a consistent therapeutic relationship, where patients can see the same provider over time, even if virtually.

Technological Innovations and Future Directions

Telemedicine has enormous potential to transform healthcare by overcoming geographic barriers and expanding access to care. Key innovations in telemedicine are likely to be enabled by AI and machine learning.[64] These technologies can help analyze patient data, diagnose conditions, and recommend treatment plans remotely.

One major innovation is likely to be intelligent chatbots and virtual assistants. Chatbots "are automated systems that replicate user's behavior on one side of the chat communication. They are mimic systems which imitate the conversations between two individuals."[65] Chatbots powered by natural language processing can have conversational interactions with patients to collect symptoms and medical history. Advanced chatbots may one day be able to diagnose simple conditions, recommend over-the-counter treatments, or determine if a patient should seek in-person care. Virtual assistants[66] are AI-based tools that serve patients and healthcare professionals by providing reminders, offering healthcare advice, helping patients manage medications, access records, schedule appointments, learn about diseases and treatments, and more.[70]

Another innovation is remote patient monitoring through wearables and at-home devices. AI algorithms can analyze data from smartwatches, fitness trackers, and other devices to assess a patient's vital signs, activity levels, sleep patterns, etc. This can allow doctors to identify emerging health problems and intervene early on. Sensors and the Internet of Things may also enable doctors to remotely monitor recovery and care within patients' homes.

Telemedicine is also likely to leverage innovations in robotics. Robotic systems controlled by doctors can help conduct remote examinations and diagnostics. This may include palpation, auscultation of the chest, basic imaging, and more. Robots may also assist in remote surgeries in the future.

The convenience, access, improved outcomes, and potential cost savings from these technologies could accelerate telemedicine adoption. However, challenges remain around reimbursement policies, licensing/ credentialing, device integration, and patient privacy. Addressing these concerns will shape the sustainable success of telemedicine going forward. Still, telemedicine appears poised to be a transformative healthcare delivery model if key technical and regulatory challenges can be overcome.

Impact of Telemedicine on the Healthcare Workforce

The advent of telemedicine is redefining the landscape of healthcare delivery, and with it, the dynamics of the healthcare workforce are undergoing a significant transformation.

Creation of New Roles in the Healthcare Workforce

Telemedicine has led to the emergence of new professional roles within the healthcare sector.[67] For instance, telehealth coordinators and telemedicine technicians are becoming integral parts of healthcare teams. These roles involve managing the technological aspects of telemedicine services, coordinating care between patients and providers, and ensuring the smooth operation of telehealth programs. Such positions require a unique combination of healthcare knowledge and technical proficiency.

Another burgeoning role is that of telehealth nurse practitioners, who provide remote care and consultation. They must be adept in clinical assessment via digital means, requiring not just medical expertise but also a firm grasp of the telemedicine platforms.

Need for Different Skills

The shift toward telemedicine also demands a new skill set from traditional healthcare providers.[68] Beyond clinical expertise, providers must be proficient in digital communication and the use of telehealth software. They must also be capable of conveying empathy and building rapport with patients through a screen, a skill that differs significantly from in-person interactions.

Moreover, there is a growing need for data management skills[69] as telemedicine generates vast amounts of digital health data that must be securely managed and effectively integrated into patient care.

Reshaping the Healthcare Delivery Model

Telemedicine is altering the traditional patient–provider interaction model. Providers are now required to engage in remote monitoring and virtual consultations, which can increase the efficiency of healthcare delivery by enabling providers to see more patients in less time. However, this also means that providers must adapt to providing care without physical examination, relying instead on patient-reported symptoms and digital monitoring data.

This shift also has implications for medical education and training. Curricula are increasingly incorporating telemedicine competencies, teaching students how to operate in a healthcare environment where virtual interactions are commonplace.

Patient Education and Support

Patient education and support are fundamental components in the effective deployment of telemedicine technologies.[70] As telemedicine continues to grow, ensuring that patients are well informed about how to use these technologies is crucial for enhancing engagement and improving health outcomes. This section outlines strategies to educate patients about telemedicine, fostering a collaborative and informed patient–provider relationship in a virtual healthcare environment.

Intuitive Onboarding Processes

The onboarding process is a patient's first introduction to telemedicine technology, and it should be as intuitive as possible.[71] Simple step-by-step guides, whether in written, video, or infographic format, can assist patients in setting up the hardware and software required for telemedicine consultations. For instance, a series of short, easy-to-understand tutorial videos that guide patients through setting up an account, testing their camera and microphone, and entering a virtual waiting room can demystify the process.

Accessible Educational Materials

Healthcare providers should offer accessible educational materials tailored to diverse literacy levels and languages.[72] These materials should cover not only how to use telemedicine technologies but also what to expect during a telemedicine visit, how to prepare for a consultation, and how to follow up afterward. Brochures, FAQs, and website resources can serve as permanent references for patients to access at their convenience.

Personalized Training Sessions

Personalized training sessions can be an effective way to educate patients, particularly for those less comfortable with technology. This could be done through one-on-one walk-throughs via phone or video call before the first telemedicine appointment. An even better technique would be an in-office "at-the-elbow" training with nurses or office staff. For groups that may need additional support, such as senior citizens, dedicated workshops can be organized by healthcare facilities or community centers.

Support Hotlines and Help Desks

Providing patients with access to support hotlines or help desks where they can ask questions or resolve technical issues is essential.[73] This support should be readily available, especially during the initial phases of a patient's experience with telemedicine.

Incorporating Feedback Mechanisms

Feedback mechanisms allow patients to report back on their experience with telemedicine technologies. This not only empowers patients but also provides healthcare providers with valuable insights into potential areas for improvement in their telemedicine offerings.

Continuous Follow-Ups and Reinforcement

Patient education on telemedicine should not be a one-time effort. Continuous follow-ups and reinforcement through regular communication can help keep patients informed about updates and best practices. Email newsletters, text message reminders, and social media posts are tools that can be used for ongoing patient education.

Fostering a Community of Users

A virtual community is a social network formed or facilitated through electronic media,[74] and these can be led by a professional, or exist as peer-to-peer forums. Creating a community of telemedicine users, such as online forums or virtual patient groups, can provide peer support and encourage the exchange of tips and advice. This can be particularly helpful for chronic disease management, where patients can learn from each other's experiences in using telemedicine for their care.

Global Perspective

Telemedicine has emerged as a global force in healthcare, providing innovative solutions to traditional healthcare delivery challenges. Its implementation and impact vary widely across different countries, influenced by factors such as technological infrastructure, healthcare policies, and socioeconomic conditions. This section explores the global perspective on telemedicine, highlighting the diverse ways it is being implemented around the world and the impact it is having on global health.

Developed Countries: Expansion and Integration

In developed countries, telemedicine is often seen as an extension of the existing healthcare system, enhancing access and convenience for patients. For instance, in the United States, telemedicine has been rapidly adopted due to its potential to reduce costs and extend care to rural areas. Insurance companies have begun to recognize telemedicine visits, and many states have passed parity laws requiring them to reimburse telemedicine services at the same rate as in-person visits.

In European nations, such as the United Kingdom and Sweden, telemedicine has been integrated into national health services. The United Kingdom's National Health Service (NHS) offers digital services and virtual consultations as part of its long-term plan to make healthcare more accessible.[75] Similarly, Sweden has been a pioneer in e-health, with digitalization being a key part of its healthcare strategy, aiming for the most efficient healthcare system in the world by 2025.[76]

Emerging Economies: Bridging Gaps

Emerging economies have embraced telemedicine to bridge significant healthcare gaps. For example, in India, the doctor-to-population ratio is 0.62:1,000, while the World Health Organization (WHO) recommends a doctor-to-population ratio of 1:1,000.[77] In India, the government's "Digital India" campaign has bolstered the adoption of telemedicine, particularly in rural areas where there is a shortage of doctors.[78] The eSanjeevani platform[79] is an excellent example of a state-sponsored telemedicine service that is making strides in providing accessible care to remote locations.

Brazil has also seen growth in telemedicine, especially during the COVID-19 pandemic. The country's Unified Health System (SUS) has been utilizing telemedicine to provide continuity of care, even in the Amazonian regions where healthcare facilities are sparse.[80]

Low-Income Countries: Overcoming Challenges

In low-income countries, telemedicine often faces significant challenges due to limited infrastructure and resources.[81] However, there are successful examples where telemedicine has made considerable impacts. In African countries, such as Rwanda,[82] telemedicine programs have been developed to offer remote diagnosis and treatment in partnership with international organizations and local governments.[83] These programs often focus on specific health issues, such as infectious diseases or maternal health, providing specialized care that would otherwise be unavailable.

Unique Models: Innovation and Adaptation

Some countries have developed unique telemedicine models tailored to their specific needs. Israel's telehealth services are advanced, with a focus on innovation, providing services such as remote monitoring for chronic conditions and a national telemedicine network connecting major hospitals and clinics.[84,85]

In China, internet hospitals are an emerging concept where patients can receive comprehensive healthcare services online. This initiative expands the reach of healthcare services, especially to the aging population and those in less accessible regions.[86]

Challenges and Considerations

While telemedicine's global impact is generally positive, there are challenges to consider. These include ensuring data privacy and security across different legal jurisdictions, addressing the digital divide within and between countries, and maintaining quality and standards of care. Additionally, cultural and language barriers can affect the implementation and acceptance of telemedicine services.

Conclusion

In conclusion, telemedicine stands as a testament to the ingenuity and adaptability of healthcare in the digital age. It transcends geographical boundaries, democratizes access to healthcare, and presents innovative solutions to age-old challenges of care delivery. As this chapter has explored, the successful implementation of telemedicine hinges on a multitude of factors, from technological infrastructure and regulatory environments to provider training and patient education. The global perspective on telemedicine illustrates not only its potential to revolutionize healthcare delivery but also the need for a collaborative, cross-border approach in addressing the accompanying challenges. Moving forward, we must continue to refine telemedicine practices, ensuring that they remain patient-centered, secure, and equitable. The journey of telemedicine is far from complete, but it promises a future where quality healthcare is within reach for every individual, regardless of where they live.

References

1. Palozzi G, Schettini I, Chirico A. Enhancing the sustainable goal of access to healthcare: findings from a literature review on telemedicine employment in rural areas. *Sustainability*. 2020 Jan;12(8):3318.
2. Pool J, Akhlaghpour S, Fatehi F, Gray LC. Data privacy concerns and use of telehealth in the aged care context: an integrative review and research agenda. *Int J Med Inform*. 2022;160:104707. doi:10.1016/j.ijmedinf.2022.104707.
3. American Medical Association. 2021 Telehealth Survey Report. 2022. https://www.ama-assn.org/system/files/telehealth-survey-report.pdf. Accessed 2023 Dec 11.
4. Standage T. *The Victorian Internet: The Remarkable Story of the Telegraph and the Nineteenth Century's On-Line Pioneers*. New York: Walker and Company; 1998.
5. Bashshur RL, Shannon GW, Sapci H. Telemedicine evaluation. *Telemed J E Health*. 2005;11(3):296–316. doi:10.1089/tmj.2005.11.296.
6. Zundel KM. Telemedicine: history, applications, and impact on librarianship. *Bull Med Libr Assoc*. 1996 Jan;84(1):71–79. PMID: 8938332; PMCID: PMC226126.

7. Jagarapu J, Savani RC. A brief history of telemedicine and the evolution of teleneonatology. *Semin Perinatol*. 2021;45:151416.

8. Perednia DA, Allen A. Telemedicine technology and clinical applications. *JAMA*. 1995;273(6):483–488. doi:10.1001/jama.1995.03520300057037.

9. Link MM. *Space Medicine in Project Mercury. NASA SP-4003*. Washington: Office of Manned Space Flight, National Aeronautics and Space Administration; 1965. Accessed 2020 Nov 16.

10. Freiburger G, Holcomb M, Piper D. The STARPAHC collection: part of an archive of the history of telemedicine. *J Telemed Telecare*. 2007;13(5):221–223. doi:10.1258/135763307781458949. PMID: 17697507.

11. Wittson CL, Dutton R. A new tool in psychiatric education. *Mental Hosp*. 1955;11:35–38.

12. Wittson CL, Benschoter R. Two-way television: helping the medical centre reach out. *Am J Psychiatry*. 1972;129:624–627.

13. Krupinski EA, Antoniotti N, Bernard J. Utilization of the American Telemedicine Association's clinical practice guidelines. Telemed J E Health. 2013;19(11):846–851. doi:10.1089/tmj.2013.0027. PMID: 24050615; PMCID: PMC3810615.

14. Madsen C, Poropatich R, Koehlmoos TP. Telehealth in the military health system: impact, obstacles, and opportunities. *Mil Med*. 2023;188(Suppl 1):15–23. doi:10.1093/milmed/usac207.

15. Crowther MJ, Poropatich LR. Telemedicine in the US army: case reports from Somalia and Croatia. *Telemed J*. 1995;1(1):73–80.

16. U.S. Army. Telemedicine & Advanced Technology Research Center (TATRC). USAMRMC STRATEGIC COMMUNICATION PLAN. https://sites.duke.edu/pubpol590_05_s2019_team3/files/2019/01/MRMC_StratComm_TATRC_0116.pdf. Accessed 2023 Dec 9

17. World Health Organization. *mHealth: New Horizons for Health Through Mobile Technologies*. Geneva: World Health Organization; 2011.

18. Lemon CA, Kim J, Haraguchi D, Sud A, Branley J, Khadra MH. Maintaining continuity of care in a multidisciplinary health service by using m-health technologies to develop patient medical records. Proceedings of the International Conference on Health Informatics (ICHI); Vilamoura, Portugal; 2013 Nov 7–9. p. 84–87.

19. Steinhubl SR, Muse ED, Topol EJ. The emerging field of mobile health. *Sci Transl Med*. 2015;7(283):283rv3. doi:10.1126/scitranslmed.aaa3487.

20. Litan RE. *Vital Signs Via Broadband: Remote Health Monitoring Transmits Savings, Enhances Lives*. [place unknown]: Better Health Care Together; 2008.

21. Moss P, Ascari A, Bakshi A, Grijpink F. *mHealth: A New Vision for Healthcare*. New York: McKinsey & Company; 2010.

22. MAHSO. National Planning Strategy — Telehealth. MAHSO. 2021. https://www.va.gov/AIRCOMMISSIONREPORT/docs/Telehealth-National-Planning-Strategy.pdf. Accessed 2024 Mar 21.

23. Scott Kruse C, Karem P, Shifflett K, Vegi L, Ravi K, Brooks M. Evaluating barriers to adopting telemedicine worldwide: a systematic review. *J Telemed Telecare*. 2018;24(1):4–12. doi:10.1177/1357633X16674087.

24. Bestsennyy O, Gilbert G, Harris A, Rost J. *Telehealth: A Quarter-Trillion-Dollar Post-COVID-19 Reality?* New York: McKinsey & Company; 2021 May 29. https://www.mckinsey.com/industries/healthcare-systems-and-services/our-insights/telehealth-a-quarter-trillion-dollar-post-covid-19-reality.

25. Koonin LM, Hoots B, Tsang CA, Leroy Z, Farris K, Jolly T, et al. Trends in the use of telehealth during the emergence of the COVID-19 pandemic — United States, January-March 2020. *MMWR Morb Mortal Wkly Rep*. 2020 Oct 30;69(43):1595–1599. doi:10.15585/mmwr.mm6943n3. Erratum in: *MMWR Morb Mortal Wkly Rep*. 2020 Nov 13;69(45):1711. PMID: 33119561; PMCID: PMC7641006.

26. Bhaskar S, Bradley S, Chattu VK, Adisesh A, Nurtazina A, Kyrykbayeva S, et al. Telemedicine across the globe-position paper from the COVID-19 pandemic health system resilience PROGRAM (REPROGRAM) international consortium (Part 1). *Front Public Health*. 2020 Oct 16;8:556720. doi:10.3389/fpubh.2020.556720. PMID: 33178656; PMCID: PMC7596287.

27. Lin C, Pham H, Zhu Y, Clingan SE, Lin LA, Murphy SM, et al. Telemedicine along the cascade of care for substance use disorders during the COVID-19 pandemic in the United States. *Drug Alcohol Depend*. 2023 Jan 1;242:109711. doi:10.1016/j.drugalcdep.2022.109711. Epub 2022 Nov 23. PMID: 36462230; PMCID: PMC9683518.

28. CMS.gov. President Trump expands telehealth benefits for Medicare beneficiaries during COVID-19 outbreak. 2020. https://www.cms.gov/newsroom/press-releases/president-trump-expands-telehealth-benefits-medicare-beneficiaries-during-covid-19-outbreak. Accessed 2023 Dec 10.

29. Foley & Lardner LLP. Congress Wows with Medicare Telehealth Parity Act of 2015, But Will It Succeed? FOLEY. 2015. https://www.foley.com/insights/publications/2015/07/congress-wows-with-medicare-telehealth-parity-act/. Accessed 2024 Mar 24.

30. Jercich K. CONNECT for Health Act Reintroduced, Would Expand Telehealth Access. Health Care IT News. 2024. https://www.healthcareitnews.

com/news/connect-health-act-reintroduced-would-expand-telehealth-access. Accessed 2023 Dec 10.

31. CMS.gov. Coronavirus & Flexibilities. https://www.cms.gov/coronavirus-waivers. Accessed 2023 Dec 10.

32. Telehealth.HHS.gov. Telehealth Policy Changes After the COVID-19 Public Health Emergency. 2023. https://telehealth.hhs.gov/providers/telehealth-policy/policy-changes-after-the-covid-19-public-health-emergency. Accessed 2023 Dec 10.

33. U.S. Department of Health and Human Services. Notification of Enforcement Discretion for Telehealth Remote Communications During the COVID-19 Nationwide Public Health Emergency. 2021. https://www.hhs.gov/hipaa/for-professionals/special-topics/emergency-preparedness/notification-enforce-ment-discretion-telehealth/index.html. Accessed 2023 Dec 10.

34. U.S. Department of Health and Human Services. HIPAA and Telehealth. 2023. https://www.hhs.gov/hipaa/for-professionals/special-topics/telehealth/index.html. Accessed 2023 Dec 10.

35. U.S. Department of Health and Human Services. Internet access for rural telehealth patients and providers. Telehealth.HHS.gov. https://telehealth.hhs.gov/providers/best-practice-guides/telehealth-for-rural-areas/access-to-inter-net-and-other-telehealth-resources#:~:text=telehealth%20technology%20challenges-,Internet%20access%20for%20rural%20telehealth%20patients%20and%20providers,strong%20cell%20signal%2C%20if%20available. Accessed 2024 Dec 5.

36. U.S. Department of Agriculture. Hurricane resources. USDA. https://www.fcc.gov/reports-research/reports/broadband-progress-reports/fourteenth-broadbanddeployment-report accessed 12/5/24. Accessed 2024 Dec 5.

37. U.S. Department of Agriculture. e-Connectivity for All Rural Americans Is a Modern-Day Necessity. https://www.usda.gov/broadband#:~:text=Unfortunately%2C%2022.3%20percent%20of%20Americans,by%20the%20Federal%20Communications%20Commission. Accessed 2023 Dec 11.

38. Technology Use Among Seniors. Pew Research Center. 2017. https://www.pewresearch.org/internet/2017/05/17/technology-use-among-seniors/#:~:text=Younger%20seniors%20use%20the%20internet,30%25). Accessed 2024 Jun 14.

39. NIHCM Foundation. Rural Health: Addressing Barriers to Care. 2023. https://nihcm.org/publications/rural-health-addressing-barriers-to-care.

40. Crowley MJ, Tarkington PE, Bosworth HB, Jeffreys AS, Coffman CJ, Maciejewski ML, et al. Effect of a comprehensive telehealth intervention vs telemonitoring and care coordination in patients with persistently poor type

2 diabetes control: a randomized clinical trial. *JAMA Intern Med.* 2022;182(9):943–952. doi:10.1001/jamainternmed.2022.2947.

41. Haleem A, Javaid M, Singh RP, Suman R. Telemedicine for healthcare: Capabilities, features, barriers, and applications. *Sens Int.* 2021;2:100117. doi:10.1016/j.sintl.2021.100117. Epub 2021 Jul 24. PMID: 34806053; PMCID: PMC8590973.

42. Serag-Bolos ES, Barbarello Andrews L, Beall J, Lempicki KA, Miranda AC, Motycka C, et al. Clinical skills development in the virtual learning environment: adapting to a new world. In: Ford C, Garza K, editors. *Handbook of Research on Updating and Innovating Health Professions Education: Post-Pandemic Perspectives.* Hershey: IGI-Global; 2022. p. 265–297. doi:10.4018/978-1-7998-7623-6.ch012.

43. Greenhalgh T, Koh GCH, Car J. Covid-19: a remote assessment in primary care. *BMJ.* 2020;368:m1182.

44. Jalali MS, Landman A, Gordon WJ. Telemedicine, privacy, and information security in the age of COVID 19. *J Am Med Inform Assoc.* 2021 Mar 1;28(3):671–672. doi:10.1093/jamia/ocaa310. PMID: 33325533; PMCID: PMC7798938.

45. Raposo VL. Telemedicine: the legal framework (or the lack of it) in Europe. *GMS Health Technol Assess.* 2016 Aug 16;12:Doc03. doi:10.3205/hta000126. PMID: 27579146; PMCID: PMC4987488.

46. Holčapek T, Šolc M, Šustek P. Telemedicine and the standard of care: a call for a new approach? *Front Public Health.* 2023 May 4;11: 1184971. doi:10.3389/fpubh.2023.1184971. PMID: 37213629; PMCID: PMC10192621.

47. Nittari G, Khuman R, Baldoni S, Pallotta G, Battineni G, Sirignano A, et al. Telemedicine practice: review of the current ethical and legal challenges. *Telemed J E Health.* 2020 Dec;26(12):1427–1437. doi:10.1089/ tmj.2019.0158. Epub 2020 Feb 12. PMID: 32049608; PMCID: PMC7757597.

48. Hilty DM, Crawford A, Teshima J, Nasatir-Hilty SE, Luo J, Chisler LSM, et al. Mobile health and cultural competencies as a foundation for telehealth care: scoping review. *J Technol Behav Sci.* 2021;6:197–230. doi:10.1007/ s41347-020-00180-5.

49. Jensen E, Jones N, Rabe M, Pratt B, Medina L, Orozco K, et al. The Chance that Two People Chosen at Random Are of Different Race or Ethnicity Groups Has Increased Since 2010. United States Census Bureau. 2023. https://www.census.gov/library/stories/2021/08/2020-united-states-population-more-racially-ethnically-diverse-than-2010.html. Accessed 2023 Dec 10.

50. Prasad A, Brewster R, Rajasekaran D, Rajasekaran K. Preparing for telemedicine visits: guidelines and setup. *Front Med (Lausanne)*. 2020 Nov 25; 7:600794. doi:10.3389/fmed.2020.600794. PMID: 33324665; PMCID: PMC7724018.

51. AMA. Follow this Checklist to Brighten Your Telehealth Presence. 2023. https://www.ama-assn.org/practice-management/digital/follow-checklist-brighten-your-telehealth-presence. Accessed 2023 Dec 10.

52. Telehealth Competencies. AAMC. 2024. https://www.aamc.org/data-reports/report/telehealth-competencies. Accessed 2023 Dec 10.

53. Taskforce on Telehealth Policy (TTP): Findings and Recommendations. NCQA. 2020. https://www.ncqa.org/programs/data-and-information-technology/telehealth/taskforce-on-telehealth-policy/taskforce-on-telehealth-policy-ttp-findings-and-recommendations/. Accessed 2023 Dec 11.

54. Demaerschalk BM, Hollander JE, Krupinski E, Scott J, Albert D, Bobokalonova Z, et al. Quality frameworks for virtual care: expert panel recommendations. *Mayo Clin Proc Innov Qual Outcomes*. 2022 Dec 29;7(1):31–44. doi:10.1016/j.mayocpiqo.2022.12.001. PMID: 36619179; PMCID: PMC9811201.

55. Ransdell LB, Greenberg ME, Isaki E, Lee A, Bettger JP, Hung G, et al. Practices for building interprofessional telehealth: report of a conference. *Int J Telerehabil*. 2021 Dec 16;13(2):e6434. doi:10.5195/ijt.2021.6434. PMID: 35646239; PMCID: PMC9098135.

56. Hall JL, McGraw D. For telehealth to succeed, privacy and security risks must be identified and addressed. *Health Aff (Millwood)*. 2014 Feb;33(2):216–221. doi:10.1377/hlthaff.2013.0997. PMID: 24493763.

57. Houser SH, Flite CA, Foster SL. Privacy and security risk factors related to telehealth services — a systematic review. *Perspect Health Inf Manag*. 2023 Jan 10;20(1):1f. PMID: 37215337; PMCID: PMC9860467.

58. BroadbandNow. FCC underestimates unserved by 50 percent. BroadbandNow. https://broadbandnow.com/research/fcc-underestimates-unserved-by-50-percent. Accessed 2024 Dec 5.

59. Van Dyk L. A review of telehealth service implementation frameworks. *Int J Environ Res Public Health*. 2014;11(2):1279–1298.

60. Choxi H, VanDerSchaaf H, Li Y, Morgan E. Telehealth and the digital divide: identifying potential care gaps in video visit use. *J Med Syst*. 2022 Jul 30;46(9):58. doi:10.1007/s10916-022-01843-x. PMID: 35906432; PMCID: PMC9361960.

61. Drake C, Lian T, Cameron B, Medynskaya K, Bosworth HB, Shah K. Understanding telemedicine's "new normal": variations in telemedicine use by specialty line and patient demographics. *Telemed J E Health*. 2022 Jan;28(1):51–59. doi:10.1089/tmj.2021.0041. Epub 2021 Mar 25. PMID: 33769092; PMCID: PMC8785715.

62. Tierney AA, Payán DD, Brown TT, Aguilera A, Shortell SM, Rodriguez HP. Telehealth use, care continuity, and quality: diabetes and hypertension care in community health centers before and during the COVID-19 pandemic. *Med Care*. 2023 Apr 1;61(Suppl 1):S62–S69. doi:10.1097/MLR.0000000000001811. Epub 2023 Mar 9. PMID: 36893420; PMCID: PMC9994572.

63. Hardcastle L, Ogbogu U. Virtual care: enhancing access or harming care? *Healthc Manage Forum*. 2020;33(6):288–292. doi:10.1177/0840470420938818.

64. Kuziemsky C, Maeder AJ, John O, Gogia SB, Basu A, Meher S, et al. Role of artificial intelligence within the telehealth domain. *Yearb Med Inform*. 2019 Aug;28(1):35–40. doi:10.1055/s-0039-1677897. Epub 2019 Apr 25. PMID: 31022750; PMCID: PMC6697552.

65. Bhirud N, Tataale S, Randive S, Nahar S. A literature review on chatbots in healthcare domain. *Int J Sci Technol Res*. 2019 July;8(07):225–231. ISSN 2277-8616.

66. World Pharma Today. The Role of Virtual Healthcare Assistants in Enhancing Telemedicine. [Cited 2024 Oct 21]. https://www.worldpharmatoday.com/news/the-role-of-virtual-healthcare-assistants-in-enhancing-telemedicine/.

67. Mrinetwork. The Rise of Telemedicine: Recruiting Top Talent in a Digital Healthcare Landscape. Mrinetwork. 2023. https://mrinetwork.com/hiring-talent-strategy/the-rise-of-telemedicine-recruiting-top-talent-in-a-digital-healthcare-landscape/#:~:text=Specialized%20Roles%3A%20Telemedicine%20has%20given,have%20skill%20for%20healthcare%20professionals.

68. Galpin K, Sikka N, King SL, Horvath KA, Shipman SA, the AAMC Telehealth Advisory Committee. Expert consensus: telehealth skills for health care professionals. *Telemed J E Health*. 2021;27(7):820–824.

69. Osterday J. Healthcare Data Management and the Future of Medicine. HTEC. 2021. https://htecgroup.com/the-increasing-importance-of-data-management-in-healthcare/.

70. Wetter D. The Importance of Patient Education in Your Telehealth Program. Health Recovery Solutions. https://www.healthrecoverysolutions.com/blog/

your-telehealth-program-the-importance-of-patient-and-clinician-education.
Accessed 2023 Dec 11.

71. Hron JD, Parsons CR, Williams LA, Harper MB, Bourgeois FC.
     Rapid implementation of an inpatient telehealth program during the
     COVID-19 pandemic. *Appl Clin Inform.* 2020 May;11(3):452–459.
     doi:10.1055/s-0040-1713635. Epub 2020 Jul 1. PMID: 32610350; PMCID:
     PMC7329373.

72. Andrulis DP, Brach C. Integrating literacy, culture, and language to improve
     health care quality for diverse populations. *Am J Health Behav.* 2007
     Sep–Oct;31(Suppl 1):S122–S133. doi:10.5555/ajhb.2007.31.supp.S122.
     PMID: 17931131; PMCID: PMC5091931.

73. Appleton R, Barnett P, Vera San Juan N, Tuudah E, Lyons N, Parker J, et al.
     Implementation strategies for telemental health: a systematic review. *BMC
     Health Serv Res.* 2023 Jan 25;23(1):78. doi:10.1186/s12913-022-08993-1.
     PMID: 36694164; PMCID: PMC9873395. Accessed 2023 Dec 11.

74. Wellman B. An electronic group is virtually a social network. In: Kiesler S,
     editor. *Cultures of the Internet.* Mahwah: Lawrence Erlbaum;1997.
     p. 170–205.

75. Brown MRD, Knight M, Peters CJ, Maleki S, Motavalli A, Nedjat-Shokouhi
     B. Digital outpatient health solutions as a vehicle to improve healthcare sus-
     tainability — a United Kingdom focused policy and practice perspective.
     Front Digit Health. 2023 Sep 26;5:1242896. doi:10.3389/fdgth.2023.1242896.
     PMID: 37829594; PMCID: PMC10566364.

76. Tikkanen R, Osborn R, Mossialos E, Djordjevic A, Wharton GA. International
     Health Care System Profiles Sweden. The Commonwealth Fund. 2020.
     https://www.commonwealthfund.org/international-health-policy-center/
     countries/sweden.

77. Doctor patient ratio in India [Internet]. 164.100.47.190; 2018. [cited
     2018 Dec 1]. http://164.100.47.190/loksabhaquestions/annex/12/AS86.pdf.
     Accessed 2023 Dec 11.

78. Chellaiyan VG, Nirupama AY, Taneja N. Telemedicine in India: where do we
     stand? *J Family Med Prim Care.* 2019 Jun;8(6):1872–1876. doi:10.4103/
     jfmpc.jfmpc_264_19. PMID: 31334148; PMCID: PMC6618173.

79. Dastidar BG, Suri S, Nagaraja VH, Jani A. A virtual bridge to Universal
     Healthcare in India. *Commun Med (Lond).* 2022 Nov 16;2(1):145.
     doi:10.1038/s43856-022-00211-7. PMID: 36385160; PMCID: PMC9667848.

80. Nunes FGD, Santos AMD, Carneiro ÂO, Fausto MCR, Cabral LMdS, de
     Almeida PF. et al. Challenges to the provision of specialized care in remote

rural municipalities in Brazil. *BMC Health Serv Res.* 2022;22(1):1386. doi:10.1186/s12913-022-08805-6.

81. Dodoo JE, Al-Samarraie H, Alzahrani AI. Telemedicine use in Sub-Saharan Africa: barriers and policy recommendations for Covid-19 and beyond. *Int J Med Inform.* 2021 Jul;151:104467. doi:10.1016/j.ijmedinf.2021.104467. Epub 2021 Apr 24. PMID: 33915421; PMCID: PMC9761083.

82. de Roodenbeke E, Lucas S, Rouzaut A, Bana F. Outreach Services as a Strategy to Increase Access to Health Workers in Remote and Rural Areas: Increasing Access to Health Workers in Rural and Remote Areas. Technical Report, No. 2. Geneva: World Health Organization; 2011.

83. Bervell B, Al-Samarraie H. A comparative review of mobile health and electronic health utilization in sub-Saharan African countries. *Soc Sci Med.* 2019;232:1–16.

84. Reicher S, Sela T, Toren O. Using telemedicine during the COVID-19 pandemic: attitudes of adult health care consumers in Israel. *Front Public Health.* 2021 May 17;9:653553. doi:10.3389/fpubh.2021.653553. PMID: 34079784; PMCID: PMC8165259.

85. Even-Zohr A, Ironi A, Ben- Itzhak R. Online health services for older adults Maccabi healthcare services. *Gerontol Geriatr.* 2017;2:1–34.

86. Han Y, Lie RK, Guo R. The internet hospital as a telehealth model in China: systematic search and content analysis. *J Med Internet Res.* 2020 Jul 29;22(7):e17995. doi:10.2196/17995. PMID: 32723721; PMCID: PMC7424477.

Chapter 3

Robots in Medicine

The word "robot" generally refers to a machine capable of carrying out a complex series of actions automatically, especially one programmable by a computer. Robots can be autonomous, semiautonomous, or remotely controlled. They are designed to perform tasks either in place of humans or in hazardous or inaccessible environments. The concept and application of robots vary widely and include industrial robots, service robots, medical robots, and more.

The origin of the word "robot" comes from the Czech word "robota," meaning "forced labor" or "servitude." It was first used to describe a fictional humanoid in the 1920 play "R.U.R." ("Rossum's Universal Robots") by Karel Čapek. Since then, the definition has evolved to encompass a broad range of automated machines, from simple mechanical devices to complex AI-driven entities capable of learning and decision-making.

Robots were typically used to accomplish tasks that were too dirty, dangerous, or distant for humans. Examples include applications in manufacturing, mining, and the defense industry. In healthcare today, robots are used to increase control and consistency of procedures and to provide capabilities that caregivers do not have.

The term "medical robot" encompasses diverse robotic systems designed for medical interventions. These robots vary from autonomous, capable of functioning with minimal human intervention, to semiautonomous, requiring significant human control or guidance.

Autonomous vs Semiautonomous Robots

Autonomous robots in medicine operate independently within a predefined scope; these robots can perform medical tasks without human intervention but within a limited and clearly defined range of operations. This limitation is essential for safety and efficacy. A notable example is the CyberKnife,[1] a robotic radiosurgery system that autonomously targets and treats tumors with high-dose radiation, as detailed by Adler et al.[2] in their 1997 study published in *Stereotactic and Functional Neurosurgery*.

In contrast, a semiautonomous surgical robot combines human control with autonomous capabilities. This means that the robot can assist the surgeon with specific tasks, but the overall control of the operation remains with the surgeon. An example of this type of robot is the da Vinci Surgical System, which requires human oversight. The surgeon controls the robot's arms while viewing a high-definition 3D surgical site image.[3]

Medical Robots by Application

Medical robots can also be categorized based on their applications. These applications include surgical robots, rehabilitation robots, telepresence robots, and telesurgery robots.

Surgical robots, exemplified by systems like the da Vinci Surgical System, have significantly advanced medical technology, particularly in performing minimally invasive surgeries. These robots, controlled by surgeons, offer enhanced precision, control, and flexibility, crucial for complex surgeries. Their ability to perform intricate movements in confined spaces surpasses human capabilities, reducing the risk of surgical errors.

A vital advantage of these robots is their design for minimally invasive procedures, leading to smaller incisions, less pain, and quicker patient recovery times. This benefit is particularly notable in laparoscopic surgeries. Additionally, they provide magnified, high-definition, 3D views of the surgical site, offering surgeons a clarity of field and detailed perspective essential in delicate operations such as neurosurgery or microsurgery.

Ergonomics is another important aspect of these systems. For example, in the da Vinci system, surgeons operate seated at a console, reducing physical strain during lengthy procedures. Furthermore, integrating machine learning and advanced data processing in robotic surgery enhances precision and effectiveness, with AI algorithms providing data-driven insights and augmenting the surgeon's skills.

Studies, including those published in the *Journal of the American Medical Association*, have shown positive patient outcomes with robotic surgery.[4,5] These include a 52% reduction in readmission rates and a 77% decrease in the incidence of blood clots such as deep vein thrombosis and pulmonary embolisms compared to open surgery. These findings highlight the advantages of robotic surgery in improving patient safety and reducing complications.

The widespread adoption of surgical robots, such as the da Vinci system, is evident with over 5,500 installations worldwide and usage in over 12 million surgeries. The United States leads in robotic surgeries, particularly in general surgery. However, concerns about cost-effectiveness persist, as robotic surgery can be more expensive than traditional methods. The initial learning curve for surgical teams is also a consideration, though outcomes tend to improve with experience and technological advancements.

Regarding hospital efficiency and patient safety, robot-assisted surgery (RAS) has made a significant impact. RAS contributes to shorter hospital stays and minimizes tissue damage and bleeding, leading to fewer complications and faster healing.[6] This efficiency reduces healthcare costs and improves long-term patient outcomes, including reduced pain and improved quality of life. While initial investments in RAS are high, the long-term benefits for hospitals and patients are substantial, with ongoing technological advancements likely to increase its prevalence in the surgical field.

Surgical Robots

A surgical robot is a type of semiautonomous robotic system specifically designed to assist in performing surgical procedures. These robots are typically controlled by surgeons and facilitate the precision, control, and flexibility required during complex surgeries.

Since their introduction in 2000,[7] surgical robots have represented a significant advancement in medical technology, enhancing surgeons' capabilities in various ways. Robotic surgery is increasingly prevalent globally. Currently, over 50,000 surgeons are certified in this technique, and upward of 6,730 surgical robots are in use across 69 different countries.[8,9]

Robotic-assisted surgery (RAS) has been adopted across a wide range of surgical subspecialties,[10] receiving approval for use in urology, gynecology, cardiothoracic surgery, general surgery, and otolaryngology. In 2023, robotic surgery will account for more than 15% of all general surgical procedures.[4] The most common procedure performed with a robotic system is the laparoscopic cholecystectomy.[4]

These robots are known for their enhanced precision and control. The robotic arms can surpass the limitations of human hands because they can rotate and maneuver in ways that human hands cannot. The advantages of manipulation involve articulated instruments, offering seven degrees of freedom in movement, counteracting the fulcrum effect, filtering out tremors, and enabling the scaling of movements.[11,12]

The delicate movements of robotic arms, which minimize tissue damage and bleeding, lead to fewer complications and faster healing.[13,14] This is particularly evident in procedures requiring intricate movements in confined spaces. They can perform repetitive and precise tasks without fatigue. These capabilities can help to reduce the risk of surgical errors. This reduces the need for blood transfusions and additional surgeries, ultimately improving patient safety and lowering healthcare costs.[15]

Furthermore, surgical robots often provide well-lit, magnified, high-definition, and 3D views of the surgical site. This advanced visualization surpasses traditional methods, offering surgeons a more precise and detailed view of the pivotal operating area in delicate surgeries such as neurosurgery or microsurgery.

Ergonomics is also a significant consideration in the design of surgical robots. These systems can reduce surgeon fatigue by offering more comfortable and ergonomic ways to perform surgeries, which is especially beneficial during lengthy procedures. Indeed, surgeons reported substantially less physical discomfort when using the robotic platform than traditional laparoscopic and open surgery.[16] The ergonomic design of these robotic surgical systems is evident in the da Vinci system, where surgeons can operate from a seated position at a console, with their head up looking at a display rather than with their necks flexed, reducing physical strain.

In addition, survey data were evaluated, indicating that, regardless of surgeons' experience, tasks completed on the robotic platform involved less cognitive workload than the same tasks completed with laparoscopy.[17] Less physical and mental fatigue should allow surgeons to perform at a higher skill level for longer durations of time, and it may even extend their careers.

Lastly, integrating machine learning and advanced data processing is a frontier in robotic surgery. Advanced systems can integrate with preoperative imaging data and utilize machine learning algorithms to assist in planning and executing surgical procedures, enhancing the overall precision and effectiveness of surgeries.

Studies of robotic surgical procedures have generally shown positive patient outcomes[5,18] and high levels of patient satisfaction, especially in terms of reduced pain, shorter hospital stays,[19] and quicker return to normal activities.[20] The advantages of robotic-assisted surgery are well documented in both general surgery and surgical oncology. Compared to traditional laparoscopic techniques, patients in these fields enjoy benefits that traditional laparoscopic techniques often struggle to match. Patients reap the rewards of a gentler touch, thanks to robotic procedures' minimally invasive nature. This translates to less tissue manipulation and, consequently, reduced postoperative pain.[21] The benefits go beyond immediate comfort, however. Surgeons adept in robotic techniques can tackle complex procedures laparoscopically, significantly lowering the open conversion rate and the extended recovery time.[22] This means shorter hospital stays and a quicker return to the familiar rhythms of life for patients.

For instance, a study published in the *Journal of the American Medical Association* found that robotic-assisted surgeries could reduce patient hospital stays by 21% compared to traditional methods.[23] This comparison underscores the significant advantages of robotic surgery over conventional open surgical procedures.

Robotic surgery can result in fewer complications.[24] For example, a recent study featured in the *Journal of the American Medical Association*[25] reports a notable decrease in readmission rates, by 52%, for patients undergoing robotic surgery compared to those who had open surgery. Additionally, the study highlights a remarkable reduction, by 77%, in the incidence of blood clots, including deep vein thrombosis and pulmonary embolisms. These conditions are known for their profound impact on health and morbidity. Also, the journal *Surgery* recently reported on a national study of abdominal surgeries comparing outcomes in RAS to those in laparoscopic surgery. It showed a 2.2% reduction in complications in the RAS surgery.[26]

All told, robotic-assisted surgery promises a smoother, faster road to recovery, a welcome advantage in the often-daunting landscape of general and oncological surgery.

Surgical robots like the da Vinci Surgical System stand at the forefront of this technological revolution. These systems have been widely adopted for various procedures, including urologic, gynecologic, and cardiac surgery. Intuitive Surgical, the manufacturer of the da Vinci systems, reported that over 5,500 da Vinci Surgical Systems were installed worldwide.[27] The da Vinci system has been used in over 12 million surgeries globally,[28] indicating its effectiveness and global adoption. The United States now performs more robotic surgeries than anywhere else, with the majority being in general surgery.[29]

Surgical Robots and AI

Integrating AI and machine learning with medical robotics opens new frontiers in personalized and precision medicine. AI algorithms are enhancing the capabilities of surgical robots by providing data-driven insights and augmenting the surgeon's skills.

AI systems can rapidly process extensive datasets, a capability that far exceeds human limitations. This feature enables surgical robots to assimilate knowledge from thousands of recorded surgeries, offering a comprehensive learning tool for surgeons at various stages of their careers. This process is reminiscent of how Google's DeepMind AI, AlphaGo, mastered the game of Go by analyzing millions of expert moves.[30]

In identifying new trends, AI excels in sifting through global surgical data to uncover emerging patterns and techniques. This could lead to the standardization of surgical practices globally, much like AlphaGo's development of unprecedented strategies in Go.

AI also plays a crucial role in alleviating surgeons' cognitive and physical stress. By aiding in surgical planning, tool selection, real-time guidance, and operation monitoring, AI streamlines surgical procedures, enhancing efficiency and reducing surgeons' strain. This application of AI is akin to the Flyways[31] system used by Alaska Airlines, which optimizes flight paths, increases safety, and eases the cognitive load on pilots and air traffic controllers, showcasing AI's ability to boost efficiency and minimize stress.

Furthermore, AI is poised to transform surgical care, particularly in making advanced surgical techniques more accessible worldwide,[32] even in underserved areas. By offering preoperative planning, image analysis, and educational[33] and practical support to surgeons, regardless of the location, AI-enhanced robotic surgery can broaden the scope of surgeons' procedures, thereby improving global access to high-quality surgical care.

For example, surgical stapling is a technique used in organ removal, tissue cutting, sealing, and creating connections between structures. Achieving an effective staple line crucially depends on compressing the right amount of tissue between the staple jaws before activation. This skill, blending art with science, is traditionally acquired by surgeons through extensive hands-on practice across various cases and types of procedures.

The engineers at Intuitive have created a stapler that can measure tissue thickness in real time. The company's SureForm[34] staplers are enhanced with intelligent technology and designed to deliver more uniform and ideally formed staple lines. These staplers perform over a thousand measurements every second, making real-time adjustments during the stapling process. This technology not only ensures a consistent staple line but also minimizes tissue damage, accommodating a variety of tissue thicknesses.

Ongoing studies are focused on creating fully independent surgical systems capable of handling intricate tasks with deformable soft tissues, such as stitching and connecting intestinal tissues, in open surgery environments. Initial findings suggest that these supervised autonomous operations may surpass the effectiveness and consistency of surgeries conducted by seasoned surgeons and those assisted by robots.[35] The progress in autonomous robotic surgery indicates a promising future for enhancing surgical results and broadening access to refined surgical methods.

Challenges and Concerns

While the advantages of healthcare robotics are evident, the practical application of these technologies often needs to be improved. These gaps can lead to unique forms of harm that may not be easily correctable or monitored by human intervention.[36] For example, safety concerns, including the risk of injury or death, can occur if surgical robots unexpectedly shut down during a procedure or perform unintended actions.[37,38]

While robotic surgical platforms can enhance a surgeon's operating ability with advantages such as superior wrist articulation and magnified visualization, their lack of tactile feedback presents a significant hurdle. A study analyzing the learning curve for robotic procedures revealed that surgeons struggled to overcome the absence of the natural touch[39] (haptic feedback) they rely on, relying solely on visual cues. As a result, mastering robotic techniques can be challenging.

There are growing concerns regarding the cost-effectiveness of robotic surgery.

Implementing robotic surgery is associated with significant up-front costs in several critical areas, including acquisition cost, training, and maintenance.[40,41] The robotic platform itself is a considerable expense, easily costing between $1 and 2 million depending on the specific system and manufacturer; additional equipment can add another $500,000. Implementing robotic surgery requires significant training and adaptation for surgical teams that can exceed $100,000. The learning curve can impact the initial outcomes but tends to improve with experience and technological advancements.[42] These sophisticated machines require regular servicing and potential upgrades for peak performance. Maintenance and service contracts can cost $100,000–$200,000.

Quantifying the exact cost of implementing a surgical robot is difficult, as factors such as the surgical procedures offered, the volume of surgeries performed, and the chosen platform play a role. Studies have indicated that robotic surgery can be more expensive, with some findings suggesting that it may incur up to 25% higher costs compared to traditional laparoscopic surgery.[43,44]

A 2010 study across various surgical specialties offers some insight. They found that incorporating the robotic platform increased per-patient costs by an average of $1,600 compared to laparoscopy. The costs can exceed $3,200 if the initial acquisition cost is factored in. The cost differential can decrease with an increasing volume of robotically performed surgeries.[45,46] A more recent risk-adjusted trend analysis revealed that the cost discrepancy between laparoscopic and robotic-assisted surgery persisted and widened from $1,600 in 2010 to $2,600 in 2019.[29] Indeed, this study of surgical costs showed that regardless of the procedure type, all robotic-assisted operations had higher costs than laparoscopic operations, with average hospitalization costs for the laparoscopic cases equaling $16,000 compared with $18,300 for the robotic-assisted cases.

Additionally, the effectiveness of robotic surgery in comparison to other established surgical methods, such as conventional laparoscopic and open surgeries, has been questioned.[47,48] This is particularly relevant in procedures where the advantages of robotic surgery are not established or theoretically justified, such as inguinal hernia repairs. The rapid expansion of robotic surgery in areas lacking robust evidence to support its use or where there is minimal theoretical or clinical advantage has also raised concerns, with calls for more clinical scrutiny and regulation.[49]

Internet of Things and Medical Robotics

The Internet of Things (IoT) is significantly influencing the evolution of medical robotics, particularly in surgical applications. IoT, fundamentally, refers to a network linking uniquely identifiable physical devices that facilitate data collection, transmission, storage, and retrieval over the internet.[50,51] For example, intelligent inhaler devices are helping patients with asthma and chronic obstructive pulmonary disease (COPD).[52] Smart inhalers are equipped with sensors that track the usage of the medication.

They can record the time and place of each dose and sync this data with a smartphone app. This technology helps ensure patient adherence to medicines, monitor the frequency of use, and identify environmental triggers for asthma attacks.

IoT plays a pivotal role in enhancing data integration and analysis. By allowing medical robots to access comprehensive patient data, IoT can enable, for example, a more informed and precise surgical procedure.[53] This integration is not just about data volume but also about the quality and relevance of data, which is crucial for tailoring robotic-assisted surgeries to individual patient needs.

Remote operation and telemedicine represent another significant application of IoT in surgical robotics.[54] This aspect of IoT is particularly transformative, making high-quality care accessible in remote or underserved areas. However, it also brings to the fore the need for robust network infrastructures, especially in regions where connectivity is unreliable. The dependence on stable internet connections for remote surgeries poses a limitation that needs addressing for this technology to reach its full potential.

IoT-facilitated predictive maintenance of medical robots ensures operational efficiency and reduces equipment downtime. This aspect is crucial for healthcare settings where equipment availability directly impacts patient care. IoT-enabled predictive maintenance can preemptively identify potential issues, allowing for timely interventions before critical failures occur.

In training and simulation, IoT-connected robots provide real-time data and feedback, significantly enhancing the skills of medical professionals. This application is about improving technical skills and understanding patient-specific scenarios, which can be simulated more accurately with IoT data integration. Customized prosthetics and implants, created based on specific patient data gathered through IoT-connected devices, exemplify the personalized approach enabled by this technology.

The integration of IoT in pharmacy automation systems is a practical example of its broader applications. Real-time inventory tracking and enhanced medication management facilitated by IoT improve efficiency and patient safety by reducing errors in medication dispensing.

Despite these advancements, the field faces several challenges. The significant concerns center around the system's reliability and robustness and the data transmission's security.[55] Also, the complexity of healthcare data security and privacy concerns must be addressed. Ensuring the integrity and confidentiality of patient data in an IoT-enabled environment is a critical issue that requires ongoing attention and innovative solutions.[56]

Integrating IoT with surgical robotics requires a careful balance between innovation and patient safety. Ethical considerations are paramount for patient autonomy and consent in an increasingly automated healthcare environment. Additionally, the economic implications of adopting such advanced technologies must be considered, especially regarding accessibility and equity in healthcare.

Rehabilitation Robots

Rehabilitation robots are specialized technology designed to aid individuals recovering from physical injuries, surgeries, or neurological disorders.

Robot-assisted rehabilitation has been widely shown to enhance functional recovery, such as gait and upper limb function, for patients suffering from conditions such as traumatic brain injury (TBI), spinal cord injuries (SCIs), stroke, cerebral palsy, Parkinson's disease, and multiple sclerosis.[57,58] These robots are increasingly used in therapeutic settings to assist, enhance, and document rehabilitation.

The term rehabilitation robotics primarily encompasses two main types of robots: therapeutic robots and assistive robots. Each type plays a distinct role in the rehabilitation process.

Therapeutic Robots

These robots are used in the active rehabilitation process. They are designed to facilitate motor recovery and are often used in the rehabilitation of patients who have suffered from strokes, SCIs, or other conditions that affect motor function. Therapeutic robots provide repetitive, controlled, and intensive training, which is essential for neuroplasticity and recovery of motor skills. A key benefit of rehabilitation robots is their ability to facilitate repetitive and consistent movements, essential in rehabilitation exercises aimed at regaining muscle strength and motor function. These robots ensure that such tasks are performed consistently and precisely.

These robots are particularly beneficial for patients with limited mobility or strength, helping them perform movements they otherwise couldn't. As patients regain strength, these robots can also provide resistance, adding challenge and promoting muscle development. Their adaptability is another significant feature, being programmable and adjustable to meet the evolving needs of individual patients. This ensures a highly personalized and effective rehabilitation process.

An example of a therapeutic rehabilitation robot is the Lokomat, a robotic gait training device used in the rehabilitation of walking abilities. The Lokomat has improved the rehabilitation process for stroke patients, enhancing the efficiency of physical therapy, as supported by Dobkin's[59] study in *Lancet Neurology*. It consists of a robotic exoskeleton and a treadmill, programmable to move the patient's legs in a specific gait pattern and adjustable in speed and incline.

Assistive Robots

Assistive robots are those that can physically assist or assess patients to aid in achieving goals.[60] They are engineered to support individuals who face challenges with motor functions, mobility, or dexterity, enabling them to carry out daily activities more independently. These devices play a crucial role in enhancing the quality of life and autonomy for users, especially those with severe motor impairments where the potential for recovery is limited.[61,62] By assisting in everyday tasks, these robots provide significant benefits in terms of independence and overall well-being. They range from simple robotic arms that help with feeding and personal care to more complex systems such as exoskeletons that assist with walking. An example is the ReWalk exoskeleton, which has a semirigid structure that can assist the knee and hip of adults with partial and complete mobility impairments.[63] It enables individuals with SCIs to stand, walk, and climb stairs.[64]

Both types of rehabilitation robots are crucial in modern rehabilitative care, offering enhanced opportunities for recovery and independence.

In terms of feedback and monitoring, rehabilitation robots excel by providing real-time feedback to both patients and therapists.[65] Equipped with advanced sensors, they monitor and record various performance metrics, crucial for tracking progress and making informed adjustments to treatment plans. To enhance patient motivation and engagement, some robots are designed with interactive features or game-like interfaces, making therapy sessions more enjoyable and boosting patient participation.

Safety is a paramount concern in rehabilitation, and these robots contribute significantly to this area by executing movements with high precision and control.[66,67] This is crucial for patients with limited mobility or those recovering from severe injuries or neurological disorders. The robots can guide limbs through correct and safe movement patterns, reducing the risk of injury. They can be programmed to match the specific strength and mobility levels of individual patients, ensuring exercises are performed within safe limits and gradually increasing in intensity as the patient's condition improves.

The field of rehabilitation robotics is actively evolving, driven by continuous research and development.[66] This includes technological improvements and efforts to make these robots more accessible and cost-effective. Recent trends include significant innovations such as soft robots, crafted from flexible materials for a safer and more comfortable experience, and collaborative robots, or cobots, designed to work in tandem with human therapists.[68] Advances in exoskeleton technology, especially in aiding both lower and upper limb rehabilitation, have been remarkable.[69] Modern exoskeletons are increasingly lightweight and user-friendly, supporting a broader range of motion and more nuanced motor control.[70]

The integration of advanced sensors and machine learning algorithms in modern rehabilitation robots leads to more accurate monitoring of patient movements and a more responsive adaptation from the robots.[71] This tailored approach ensures that patients receive the most effective treatment for their specific needs. The COVID-19 pandemic has also spurred interest in tele-rehabilitation and robotic systems that can be used remotely or with minimal supervision.

However, the use of rehabilitation robots in the United States is not uniformly distributed across all healthcare settings or geographical areas. They are more commonly found in specialized rehabilitation centers, large hospitals, and research institutions, with less presence in smaller clinics or outpatient settings due to high costs and space requirements. Geographical variation also affects adoption, with higher usage typically seen in urban and affluent areas.

The economic aspects of rehabilitation robots include initial costs, long-term benefits, and the broader impact on healthcare systems. The initial investment is substantial, with costs for acquisition, training, integration, and maintenance. However, long-term benefits such as enhanced rehabilitation outcomes, increased efficiency, and improved patient engagement can lead to cost savings and reduced healthcare costs in the long run.

Rehabilitation robots are a growing field, offering significant benefits in patient care and therapy efficiency. Their adoption varies based on factors such as location, healthcare setting, and economic considerations. Continuous advancements in technology and research are making these robots more effective, accessible, and tailored to individual patient needs.

Telepresence Robots

Telepresence robots in healthcare, equipped with advanced video and audio communication capabilities, are revolutionizing medical care delivery.[72] These mobile, remotely operated devices enable healthcare professionals to virtually interact with patients across various settings, significantly enhancing the healthcare experience. These systems can decrease costs and inconvenience while improving patient access to medical care.

The advent of telepresence robots is underpinned by significant technological advancements, including improved robotics, enhanced telecommunication infrastructure, and sophisticated software systems. These developments have made it possible for these robots to offer reliable and efficient services in healthcare environments.

One of the primary uses of telepresence robots is in remote consultations. Healthcare professionals can virtually visit patients, engage in real-time interactions, and assess their conditions from remote locations. This is particularly beneficial in rural or underserved areas, where access to medical specialists is often limited. For example, hospitals in remote regions of Alaska have employed telepresence robots to provide timely medical consultations, greatly improving access to healthcare.[73]

In addition to facilitating remote consultations, telepresence robots enable specialists to extend their reach across multiple locations without the need for physical travel. This capability is crucial in solving the growing "care crisis" in high-income countries, where an aging population requires more healthcare services than the available skilled professionals can provide.[74]

A significant application of these robots is in patient monitoring, especially in critical care environments such as intensive care units (ICUs). A study in an ICU setting showed that the use of telepresence robots increased the amount of face-to-face time between physicians and patients and reduced the average response time to patient needs from 40 minutes to just 5 minutes.[75]

Telepresence robots also play a vital role in medical education and training. They enable medical students and trainees to virtually participate in surgeries, hospital rounds, and patient consultations. This remote participation provides valuable learning experiences that might not be available in their immediate location.

From the patient's perspective, interacting with healthcare providers through a telepresence robot often feels more engaging and personal compared to traditional communication methods such as phone calls or standard video conferencing.[76,77] However, it's important to consider the varying comfort levels with technology among different patient demographics, particularly the elderly, who may find these high-tech interactions challenging.

The InTouch Vita, also known as the RP-Vita, is a remote presence robot developed collaboratively by iRobot and InTouch Health. This innovative device exemplifies the advanced capabilities of these systems. It supports medical professionals by facilitating information exchange and improving patient care in healthcare settings.[78] It is a mobile telemedicine robot equipped with a high-definition camera, microphone, and speaker, along with ports for connecting medical devices such as stethoscopes and ultrasound imagers. Controlled remotely via a laptop or tablet, the RP-VITA allows doctors to see and hear the patient and communicate through the robot's microphone and speaker. Its use in various hospitals has expanded access to expert care, particularly in remote or resource-limited settings.

Despite these advancements, telepresence robots face challenges[79] such as dependency on stable internet connections, the learning curve associated with operating these devices, and the significant investment required for their implementation. Additionally, there are concerns about ensuring the security and privacy of patient data transmitted through these devices.

Looking into the future, telepresence robots are poised for further advancements, including integration with AI for enhanced decision-making and improved autonomous navigation systems. These developments promise to further enhance their effectiveness in healthcare delivery.

Telepresence robots represent a transformative development in healthcare, offering improved access to medical care, enhanced patient monitoring, and valuable educational opportunities. Addressing the challenges and limitations of this technology will be crucial in fully realizing its potential in the healthcare sector.

Telesurgery Robots

A telesurgery robot is an advanced robotic system that integrates robotic surgery and advanced telecommunications. They are designed to enable surgeons to perform surgical procedures from a remote location.[80] Indeed, the original intention of robotic surgery was to give surgeons the ability to perform surgery from a remote distance without touching the patient.[81] These robots are typically equipped with robotic arms and a control console, which the surgeon operates, allowing them to conduct the surgery as if they were physically present in the operating room. These consoles are connected to high-speed telecommunication networks that transfer the surgeon's input from the console to the robot at a distant location. The surgeons can replicate their hand movements with high precision and control, minimizing tremors and enhancing the accuracy required for complex surgeries. These systems typically include high-definition video and audio feeds, offering the surgeon a detailed view of the surgical site and facilitating real-time communication with the in-room medical team. Often used for minimally invasive procedures, telesurgery robots enable smaller incisions, leading to reduced patient recovery times and less postoperative pain. A significant advantage of telesurgery is its ability to overcome geographical barriers, making it especially beneficial for patients in remote or underserved areas who require immediate surgical expertise that is not locally available. An example of such a system is the da Vinci Surgical System, known for its potential in remote operations. However, the widespread implementation of telesurgery faces challenges, including increased latency times, the need for high-speed, reliable internet connections, and the complexities of coordinating across different locations and time zones.

Of interest, the first transatlantic surgery, known as the Lindbergh Operation,[82] was performed in 2001 using robotic technology, demonstrating the potential for remote surgical procedures. The surgery performed was a laparoscopic cholecystectomy, which is the surgical removal of the gallbladder. The patient was in Strasbourg, France, while the surgical team, led by Dr. Jacques Marescaux, operated the robotic system from New York City, USA. This marked the first time a surgical procedure was conducted remotely across the Atlantic Ocean.

In essence, medical robots are revolutionizing healthcare by offering new capabilities in surgery, rehabilitation, and remote care. Their increasing adoption reflects the ongoing evolution of medical technology, aiming to enhance patient care and outcomes.

Current Landscape of Medical Robotics

The field of medical robotics has seen remarkable growth and diversification, impacting various aspects of healthcare. This section delves into the prevalent robotic systems in healthcare, their adoption rates and geographical distribution, and the integration of these systems with advanced technologies such as AI, machine learning, and the IoT.

Prevalent Robotic Systems in Healthcare

Pharmacy Robots

In the realm of pharmacy, automation systems are streamlining medication dispensing and management processes. A pharmacy automation system refers to the mechanized process of handling and distributing medications in pharmacies. These systems range from simple tabletop pill counters to sophisticated software and robotic systems that manage the storage, dispensing, filling, labeling, and tracking of medications.

The primary purpose of pharmacy automation systems is to improve the efficiency and accuracy of pharmacy operations, ensuring that patients receive the correct medication in the correct dosage and format. This technology plays a crucial role in modern healthcare by streamlining the workflow in pharmacies, reducing the potential for human error, and enhancing patient safety.

Robots like the Swisslog's PillPick[83] automate the packaging, storage, and dispensing of medications, reducing errors, and improving efficiency. This system represents a significant leap in pharmacy automation technology, addressing several challenges faced in medication management.

In pharmacy operations, the impact of pharmacy robots is marked by increased accuracy and efficiency. Recent reports have highlighted that automated dispensing systems have reduced medication errors to 42%[84,85] and 78%.[86] This reduction in errors directly translates to enhanced patient safety. Furthermore, the efficiency gains from automation allow pharmacists to allocate more time to direct patient care activities.[87]

Deep Cleaning Robots

In the fast-paced environment of modern healthcare, deep cleaning is a critical but resource-intensive task, demanding considerable time and staff attention. However, the advent of medical robots, particularly those equipped for sanitization and disinfection, offers a promising solution. These robots, often utilizing ultraviolet (UV) disinfection technology, are ideally suited for this repetitive and straightforward task. By employing a UV disinfection robot, maintenance staff can be freed up to concentrate on more complex duties, such as addressing repairs or handling immediate cleaning needs such as spills.[88]

UV disinfection robots are increasingly becoming a preferred choice in healthcare facilities for their efficiency in eliminating bacteria, viruses, and other harmful microorganisms on surfaces. These robots operate by emitting a UV light that sanitizes surfaces it encounters. Their design allows them to move autonomously throughout various spaces, including rooms and corridors, ensuring a thorough disinfection process. This technology not only enhances cleaning efficiency but also contributes to a safer healthcare environment by reducing the risk of infection transmission.

The effectiveness of UV light in disinfecting surfaces has been well documented in scientific literature. A systematic review published in the *International Journal of Health Sciences* highlights that ultraviolet-C (UV-C) light is a highly effective germicidal agent, capable of inactivating microorganisms such as methicillin-resistant Staphylococcus aureus (MRSA) and vancomycin-resistant enterococci on surfaces. The study emphasizes UV-C's role as an adjunct to manual cleaning protocols, significantly enhancing infection control in healthcare settings.[89] Furthermore, the autonomous nature of these robots allows for continuous, consistent cleaning without the need for direct human intervention, making them an asset in maintaining hygiene standards in healthcare facilities.

Adoption Rates and Geographical Distribution

The adoption rates and distribution of medical robots have been steadily increasing, driven by technological advancements, growing acceptance in the medical community, and an increasing emphasis on precision and efficiency in healthcare. The United States and Europe have been at the forefront in adopting medical robotics; this has been aided by substantial investments in healthcare technology. In Asia, countries like Japan and South Korea are rapidly integrating robotics into their healthcare systems, particularly in areas such as elderly care and surgery.[90]

Integration with Other Technologies

The integration of AI and machine learning with medical robotics is opening new frontiers in personalized and precision medicine.[91] AI algorithms are enhancing the capabilities of surgical robots by providing data-driven insights and augmenting the surgeon's skills enhancing learning, introducing new methodologies, reducing stress, and expanding access to quality surgical care worldwide.[92] For example, the integration of AI in the da Vinci system is aimed at providing real-time surgical guidance and decision support.[93]

This is possible because AI systems, unlike humans, can quickly absorb and recall vast amounts of information. This capability is particularly beneficial in surgical robotics, where AI can learn from thousands of surgeries, enhancing the training and skills of surgeons at all career stages. The example of Google's AlphaGo,[94] which learned complex strategies in the game of Go from millions of moves, illustrates AI's potential to master complex tasks.

AI can also analyze global data to identify new trends and methodologies in surgery, much like AlphaGo developed novel strategies in Go. This ability to detect patterns and trends can lead to improved surgical techniques and standardized practices worldwide.

AI can streamline surgical procedures by assisting in planning, tool selection, and monitoring, thus reducing the cognitive and physical burden on surgeons.[95] This aspect is likened to the AI system Flyways used in the airline industry, which optimizes flight paths to reduce stress and increase efficiency.[96]

Significant expansion of access to surgical care is possible with AI. By integrating AI with advanced robotics, surgeons can learn from the best practices regardless of their location, potentially expanding their range of specialties and reaching a broader patient population.[97–99]

Impact of RAS on Hospital Efficiency and Patient Safety

Reduced Length of Hospital Stay

RAS often leads to shorter hospital stays compared to traditional open surgeries.[100] The minimally invasive nature of RAS results in smaller incisions, which typically heal faster and with fewer complications.[101] This faster recovery means patients can be discharged sooner, thereby freeing up hospital beds and resources for other patients.

Improved Surgical Precision and Reduced Complications

The enhanced precision of robotic systems minimizes tissue trauma during surgery. This precision reduces the likelihood of complications such as infections and excessive bleeding, which in turn decreases the need for postoperative care and readmissions. Fewer complications contribute to more efficient use of hospital resources and staff.[77,102]

Increased Throughput: With potentially shorter surgeries and quicker turnover times, RAS can increase the number of surgeries that can be performed in each time frame. This efficiency is beneficial for hospitals dealing with high patient volumes.

Enhanced Surgeon Performance and Ergonomics

RAS provides surgeons with ergonomic advantages, reducing physical strain and fatigue. This can lead to improved performance, potentially reducing the duration of surgeries and enhancing the surgeon's ability to perform complex procedures. Improved surgeon performance and comfort can indirectly contribute to hospital efficiency by optimizing surgical outcomes and reducing the likelihood of errors.

Patient Satisfaction and Hospital Reputation

Improved outcomes and patient experiences with RAS can enhance a hospital's reputation, potentially attracting more patients and skilled medical professionals. High patient satisfaction can also lead to better hospital ratings, which can be beneficial for hospital administration and funding.

Training and Skill Development

RAS offers opportunities for enhanced training and skill development for surgical teams. While there is an initial learning curve, over time, these skills can lead to more efficient surgical procedures and better patient outcomes.

Cost Implications

It's important to note that the initial investment in RAS technology is significant, and the cost-effectiveness of these systems is still a subject of ongoing research. While there are efficiency gains, they need to be balanced against the high costs of acquiring and maintaining robotic surgery systems.

Challenges and Limitations

Despite these advancements, there are challenges in the widespread adoption of medical robots.[103] The high cost of these technologies, the need for specialized training for healthcare professionals, and potential technological failures are significant considerations. Additionally, the integration of these systems into existing healthcare workflows can be complex.

Conclusion

In conclusion, medical robots have brought about substantial improvements in hospital efficiency and patient safety. Their applications in surgery, pharmacy, and patient monitoring have demonstrated tangible benefits. However, addressing the challenges related to cost, training, and integration is essential for maximizing their potential. As technology continues to advance, medical robots will likely become even more integral to healthcare delivery.

Workforce Implications

The integration of medical robots into healthcare settings has significant implications for the workforce. These implications are multifaceted, affecting various aspects of healthcare delivery, workforce dynamics, and skill requirements.

Job Redefinition and Role Shifts

The introduction of robotic technology in medical procedures is significantly redefining job roles and responsibilities within the healthcare sector. This transformation is especially pronounced in areas where tasks traditionally performed manually are becoming automated, leading to multifaceted and profound implications.

The introduction of robots in medical procedures and care can redefine job roles.[104] In the realm of surgery, the role of the surgeon is undergoing a notable transition. Surgeons are moving away from direct manual intervention to roles that often involve controlling and guiding robotic systems. This shift necessitates the development of a new skill set, including proficiency in robotic systems and an in-depth understanding of their operation and limitations. Additionally, the surgeon's role is becoming more analytical, with a focus on interpreting data provided by robotic systems to make informed decisions during procedures.

Robotic systems are also bringing about advancements in surgical precision and control, enabling surgeons to perform complex procedures with greater accuracy. This enhancement is paving the way for the development of new, minimally invasive surgical techniques that were previously unfeasible with traditional methods. Consequently, surgeons must continuously update their skills to effectively leverage these new techniques.

The roles of nurses and technicians are evolving alongside these technological advancements.[105,106] They are increasingly taking on responsibilities in the setup, operation, and maintenance of robotic systems, which requires additional training. Moreover, their roles in patient care are shifting, with a greater focus on preoperative and postoperative care as robots handle more tasks during the operation.

This technological shift in surgery also necessitates a more interdisciplinary approach to healthcare.[107] Healthcare professionals are finding themselves collaborating more closely with engineers, robotic technicians, and data scientists. This collaboration is essential for the smooth operation and integration of robotic technology in medical procedures. It requires healthcare professionals to develop not only communication skills but also an understanding of technical language to effectively work alongside these new team members.

For instance, tasks that were traditionally manual may become automated, leading to a shift in the roles and responsibilities of healthcare professionals. Surgeons, nurses, and technicians may need to adapt to working alongside robots, focusing more on monitoring and supervisory roles.[108]

Medical Education and Training

The integration of robotic technology is also influencing medical education and training.[109] Curricula are adapting to include training in robotic systems, encompassing both technical operation and decision-making aided by robotic technology. As technology evolves rapidly, continuous professional development becomes crucial for healthcare professionals to keep pace with these advancements.[110]

With these changes in roles and responsibilities come new ethical and legal considerations, particularly regarding liability in robotic surgery. Healthcare professionals must understand these aspects and how they impact their practice. Despite the increased use of technology, the importance of patient interaction remains paramount. Healthcare professionals must find a balance between their technical responsibilities and patient care, ensuring that the human element of medicine is preserved.

Training and Skill Development

There is a growing need for specialized training in robotics technology.[111] Healthcare professionals will need to acquire new skills to operate, interpret, and interact with robotic systems effectively.[112–114] This requirement spans from technical know-how to understanding the integration of robotics in patient care.

Workforce Efficiency and Productivity

Robots can enhance efficiency and productivity in healthcare settings by performing tasks more quickly and accurately than humans in certain scenarios.[115] This can lead to a more efficient allocation of human resources, where healthcare professionals can focus on patient care aspects that require human judgment and empathy.

Job Creation and Loss

The adoption of robotics in healthcare can lead to job creation in areas such as robotic maintenance, programming, and system management.[116] However, it may also lead to job displacement in roles that become automated.[105] Researchers at MIT, who have studied the effect of robots on employment, state, "Our evidence shows that robots increase productivity. They are very important for continued growth of firms, but at the same time they destroy jobs, and they reduce labor demand."[117] The net impact on employment will depend on how the healthcare sector adapts and integrates these technologies.

Ethical and Legal Considerations

With the rise of medical robots, there will be an increased need for ethical guidelines and legal frameworks addressing issues such as patient safety, data security, and liability in cases of malfunctions or errors.[118] This will require collaboration between healthcare professionals, legal experts, and policymakers.

Patient–Provider Interaction

The use of robots might alter the dynamics of patient–provider interactions. Assistive social robots are used to in the care of the elderly,[119] and while helpful are not a substitute for personal care. In her book *Alone Together: Why We Expect More from Technology and Less from Each Other*,[120] Sherry Turkle argues that social interactions with robots provide superficial emotional comfort and an ersatz intimacy. This substitute for human interaction not only deepens a patient's loneliness but also tends to infantilize them. Healthcare professionals will need to balance the technological aspects of care with the human elements, ensuring that patient communication and empathy are not compromised.

Economic Impact

The integration of medical robots into healthcare settings marks a pivotal shift toward advanced care delivery. The initial investment in these systems, while substantial and impacting budget allocations, is often offset by long-term benefits such as improved efficiency, reduced error rates, and enhanced patient outcomes.

Capital expenditure for medical robots, including surgical robots, rehabilitation robots, or pharmacy automation systems, is significant.

This cost encompasses the robot itself, necessary infrastructure modifications, training for healthcare professionals, and maintenance contracts. Implementing robotic technology also requires comprehensive training for medical staff, which can be both time consuming and expensive. Moreover, integrating these systems into existing workflows may demand significant organizational change management.

Over time, the benefits become more apparent. Robots can operate continuously, performing tasks more quickly and accurately than humans in certain contexts. For instance, pharmacy robots can dispense medications rapidly with high accuracy, reducing waiting times and allowing pharmacists to focus on more critical tasks. In surgical applications, robots provide high precision, leading to fewer complications and shorter hospital stays.

This enhanced efficiency and accuracy lead to better patient throughput. Hospitals can treat more patients with the same or even fewer resources, improving the utilization of hospital beds and facilities. Additionally, once implemented, robotic systems can be updated and scaled, potentially extending their utility beyond their initial scope. This adaptability can lead to sustained improvements in hospital operations and patient care.

Conclusion

In summary, the workforce implications of medical robots are complex and encompass changes in job roles, skill requirements, efficiency, employment patterns, ethical considerations, patient interactions, and economic impacts. These changes necessitate a proactive approach in workforce planning, training, and policy development to fully leverage the benefits of robotics in healthcare.

References

1. Kurup G. CyberKnife: a new paradigm in radiotherapy. *J Med Phys*. 2010 Apr;35(2):63–64. doi:10.4103/0971-6203.62194. PMID: 20589114; PMCID: PMC2884306.

2. Adler JR Jr, Chang SD, Murphy MJ, Doty J, Geis P, Hancock SL. The Cyberknife: a frameless robotic system for radiosurgery. *Stereotact Funct Neurosurg*. 1997;69(1-4 Pt 2):124–128. doi:10.1159/000099863. PMID: 9711744.

3. Robotic-Assisted Surgery with da Vinci Systems. Intuitive Surgical. 2024. https://www.intuitive.com/en-us/patients/da-vinci-robotic-surgery. Accessed 2023 Dec 12.

4. Sheetz KH, Claflin J, Dimick JB. Trends in the adoption of robotic surgery for common surgical procedures. *JAMA Netw Open*. 2020;3(1):e1918911. doi:10.1001/jamanetworkopen.2019.18911.

5. Shyr BU, Shyr BS, Chen SC, Chang IW, Shyr YM, Wang SE. Operative results and patient satisfaction after robotic pancreaticoduodenectomy. *Asian J Surg*. 2020;43(4):519–525. ISSN 1015–9584. doi:10.1016/j.asjsur.2019.08.012.

6. Medical Advisory Secretariat. Robotic-assisted minimally invasive surgery for gynecologic and urologic oncology: an evidence-based analysis. *Ont Health Technol Assess Ser*. 2010;10(27):1–118.

7. Hussain A, Malik A, Halim MU, Ali AM. The use of robotics in surgery: a review. *Int J Clin Pract*. 2014;68:1376–1382.

8. We Believe Minimally Invasive Care Is Life-Enhancing Care. Intuitive. 2021. https://www.intuitive.com/en/about-us/company. Accessed 2023 Dec 30.

9. Strattner. Why Strattner? 2020. http://www.strattner.com.br. Accessed 2023 Dec 30.

10. Intuitive Surgical. *Annual Report 2014*. Sunnyvale, CA: Intuitive Surgical, Inc.; 2014.

11. Wong SW, Ang ZH, Yang PF, Crowe P. Robotic colorectal surgery and ergonomics. *J Robotic Surg*. 2022;16:241–246. doi:10.1007/s11701-021-01240-5.

12. Prasad SM, Prasad SM, Maniar HS, Chu C, Schuessler RB, Damiano RJ Jr. Surgical robotics: impact of motion scaling on task performance. *J Am Coll Surg*. 2004 Dec;199(6):863–868. doi:10.1016/j.jamcollsurg.2004.08.027. PMID: 15555968.

13. Wu S-Y, Chang C-L, Chen C-I, Huang C-C. Comparison of acute and chronic surgical complications following robot-assisted, laparoscopic, and traditional open radical prostatectomy among men in Taiwan. *JAMA Netw Open*. 2021 Aug 25;4(8):e2120156. doi:10.1001/jamanetworkopen.2021.20156.

14. Maertens V, Stefan S, Rutgers M, Siddiqi N, Khan JS. Oncological outcomes of open, laparoscopic and robotic colectomy in patients with transverse colon cancer. *Tech Coloproctol.* 2022 Oct;26(10):821–830. doi:10.1007/s10151-022-02650-9. Epub 2022 Jul 8. PMID: 35804251.

15. McAlpine K, Forster AJ, Breau RH, McIsaac D, Tufts J, Mallick R, et al. Robotic surgery improves transfusion rate and perioperative outcomes using a broad implementation process and multiple surgeon learning curves. *Can Urol Assoc J.* 2019 Jun;13(6):184–189. doi:10.5489/cuaj.5527. PMID: 30407153; PMCID: PMC6570603.

16. Plerhoples TA, Hernandez-Boussard T, Wren SM. The aching surgeon: a survey of physical discomfort and symptoms following open, laparoscopic, and robotic surgery. *J Robot Surg.* 2012;6(1):65–72.

17. Lee G, Lee M, Clanton T, Marohn M. *Comprehensive Assessment of Skill-Related Physical and Cognitive Ergonomics Associated with Robotic and Traditional Laparoscopic Surgeries.* Los Angeles: Sages. https://www.sages.org/meetings/annual-meeting/abstracts-archive/comprehensive-assessment-of-skill-related-physical-and-cognitive-ergonomics-associated-with-robotic-and-traditional-laparoscopic-surgeries/. Accessed 2024 Dec 18.

18. Long E, Kew F. Patient satisfaction with robotic surgery. *J Robot Surg.* 2018 Sep;12(3):493–499. doi:10.1007/s11701-017-0772-3. Epub 2017 Dec 29. PMID: 29288373.

19. Ljungqvist O, Scott M, Fearon KC. Enhanced recovery after surgery: a review. *JAMA Surg.* 2017;152:292–298.

20. Darr C, Cheufou D, Weinreich G, Hachenberg T, Aigner C, Kampe S. Robotic thoracic surgery results in shorter hospital stay and lower postoperative pain compared to open thoracotomy: a matched pairs analysis. *Surg Endosc.* 2017 Oct;31(10):4126–4130. doi:10.1007/s00464-017-5464-6. Epub 2017 Mar 8. PMID: 28275918.

21. Sun Y, Xu H, Li Z, Han J, Song W, Wang J, et al. Robotic versus laparoscopic low anterior resection for rectal cancer: a meta-analysis. *World J Surg Oncol.* 2016;14:61.

22. Sucandy I, Rayman S, Lai EC, Tang CN, Chong Y, Efanov M, et al. International robotic, laparoscopic liver resection study group investigators. Robotic versus laparoscopic left and extended left hepatectomy: an international multicenter study propensity score-matched analysis. *Ann Surg Oncol.* 2022;29(13):8398–8406.

23. Kalata S, Thumma JR, Norton EC, Dimick JB, Sheetz KH. Comparative safety of robotic-assisted vs laparoscopic cholecystectomy. *JAMA Surg.* 2023;158(12):1303–1310. doi:10.1001/jamasurg.2023.4389.

24. Jaffray B. Minimally invasive surgery. *Arch Dis Child*. 2005;90(5): 537–542.

25. Catto JWF, Khetrapal P, Ricciardi F, Ambler G, Williams NR, Al-Hammouri T, et al. Effect of robot-assisted radical cystectomy with intracorporeal urinary diversion vs open radical cystectomy on 90-day morbidity and mortality among patients with bladder cancer: a randomized clinical trial. *JAMA*. 2022;327(21):2092–2103. doi:10.1001/jama.2022.7393.

26. Ng A, Sanaiha Y, Bakhtiyar S, Ebrahimian S, Branche C, Benharash P. National analysis of cost disparities in robotic-assisted virus laparoscopic abdominal operations. *Surgery*. 2023;173:1340–1345.

27. Intuitive Surgical. *Annual Report*. Sunnyvale, CA: Intuitive Surgical, Inc.; 2020.

28. What Makes da Vinci Robotic Surgical Systems Unique? Intuitive Surgical. 2024. https://www.intuitive.com/en-us/products-and-services/da-vinci#:~: text=What%20makes%20da%20Vinci%20robotic%20surgical%20sys tems%20unique%3F&text=For%20nearly%20three%20decades%2C%20 Da,%2Dreviewed%20in%2034%2C000%2B%20articles. Accessed 2023 Dec 12.

29. Tam V, Rogers DE, Al-Abbas A, Borrebach J, Dunn SA, Zureikat AH, et al. Robotic inguinal hernia repair: a large health system's experience with the first 300 cases and review of the literature. *J Surg Res*. 2019;235:98–104. doi:10.1016/j.jss.2018.09.070.

30. AlphaGo. Google DeepMind. https://deepmind.google/technologies/ alphago/. Accessed 2023 Dec 17.

31. Alaska Airlines. 2021. https://news.alaskaair.com/newsroom/alaska-air- lines-and-airspace-intelligence-announce-first-of-its-kind-partnership-to- optimize-air-traffic-flow-with-artificial-intelligence-and-machine-learn- ing/. Accessed 2023 Dec 17.

32. Setting the Standard in Infrastructure Solutions. Utilities One. 2024. https:// utilitiesone.com/satellite-based-remote-surgery-advancing-medical-care- from-space. Accessed 2023 Dec 17.

33. Pakkasjärvi N, Luthra T, Anand S. Artificial intelligence in surgical learn- ing. *Surgeries*. 2023;4(1):86–97. doi:10.3390/surgeries4010010.

34. Exploring New Advancements in Robotics. Intuitive. 2024. https://www. intuitive.com/en-us/about-us/newsroom/exploring-new-advancements-in- robotics. Accessed 2023 Dec 17.

35. Shademan A, Decker RS, Opfermann JD, Leonard S, Krieger A, Kim PC. Supervised autonomous robotic soft tissue surgery. *Sci Transl Med*. 2016 May 4;8(337):337ra64. doi:10.1126/scitranslmed.aad9398. PMID: 27147588.

36. Amodei D, Olah C, Steinhardt J, Christiano P, Schulman J, Mané D. Concrete problems in AI safety. arXiv preprint arXiv:1606.06565; 2016.
37. Alemzadeh H, Raman J, Leveson N, Kalbarczyk Z, Iyer RK. Adverse events in robotic surgery: a retrospective study of 14 years of FDA data. *PLoS ONE.* 2016;11(4):e0151470. doi:10.1371/journal.pone.0151470.
38. Ferrarese A, Pozzi G, Borghi F, Marano A, Delbon P, Amato B, et al. Malfunctions of robotic system in surgery: role and responsibility of surgeon in legal point of view. *Open Med.* 2016;11(1):286–291.
39. Bokhari MB, Patel CB, Ramos-Valadez DI, Ragupathi M, Haas EM. Learning curve for robotic-assisted laparoscopic colorectal surgery. *Surg Endosc.* 2011;25(3):855–860.
40. Gkegkes ID, Mamais IA, Iavazzo C. Robotics in general surgery: a systematic cost assessment. *J Minim Access Surg.* 2017 Oct–Dec;13(4):243–255. doi:10.4103/0972-9941.195565. PMID: 28000648; PMCID: PMC5607789.
41. Feldstein J, Schwander B, Roberts M, Coussons H. Cost of ownership assessment for a da Vinci robot based on US real-world data. *Int J Med Robot.* 2019 Oct;15(5):e2023. doi:10.1002/rcs.2023. Epub 2019 Jul 15. PMID: 31215714.
42. Vijayakumar A, Abdel-Rasoul M, Hekmat R, Merritt RE, D'Souza DM, Jackson GP, et al. National learning curves among robotic thoracic surgeons in the United States: quantifying the impact of procedural experience on efficiency and productivity gains. *J Thorac Cardiovasc Surg.* 2024;167:869–879. doi:10.1016/j.jtcvs.2023.07.051. Epub 2023 Aug 9. PMID: 37562675.
43. Wright JD, Ananth CV, Lewin SN, Burke WM, Lu YS, Neugut AI, et al. Robotically assisted vs laparoscopic hysterectomy among women with benign gynecologic disease. *JAMA.* 2013;309(7):689–698. doi:10.1001/jama.2013.186.
44. Jeong IG, Khandwala YS, Kim JH, Han DH, Li S, Wang Y, et al. Association of robotic-assisted vs laparoscopic radical nephrectomy with perioperative outcomes and health care costs, 2003 to 2015. *JAMA.* 2017;318(16):1561–1568. doi:10.1001/jama.2017.14586.
45. Barbash GI, Glied SA. New technology and health care costs — the case of robot-assisted surgery. *New Engl J Med.* 2010;363(8):701–704.
46. Wright JD, Ananth CV, Tergas AI, Herzog TJ, Burke WM, Lewin SN, et al. An economic analysis of robotically assisted hysterectomy. *Obstet Gynecol.* 2014;123(5):1038–1048.
47. Melamed A, Margul DJ, Chen L, Keating NL, Del Carmen MG, Yan J, et al. Survival after minimally invasive radical hysterectomy for early-stage

cervical cancer. *N Engl J Med.* 2018;379(20):1905–1914. doi:10.1056/NEJMoa1804923.

48. Ramirez PT, Frumovitz M, Pareja R, Lopez A, Vieira M, Ribeiro R, et al. Minimally invasive versus abdominal radical hysterectomy for cervical cancer. *N Engl J Med.* 2018;379(20):1895–1904. doi:10.1056/NEJMoa1806395.

49. Daniel GW, Rubens EK, McClellan M. Coverage with evidence development for Medicare beneficiaries: challenges and next steps. *JAMA Intern Med.* 2013;173(14):1281–1282. doi:10.1001/jamainternmed.2013.6793.

50. Kammüller F. Combining secure system design with risk assessment for IoT healthcare systems. *IEEE International Conference on Pervasive Computing and Communications Workshops (PerCom Workshops).* 2019;961–966. https://doi.org/10.1109/PERCOMW.2019.8730776.

51. Balakrishna S, Thirumaran M, Solanki VK. IoT sensor data integration in healthcare using semantics and machine learning approaches. *A Handbook of Internet of Things in Biomedical and Cyber Physical System.* Cham: Springer; 2020;275–300.

52. Zabczyk C, Blakey JD. The effect of connected "smart" inhalers on medication adherence. *Front Med Technol.* 2021 Aug 18;3:657321. doi:10.3389/fmedt.2021.657321. PMID: 35047916; PMCID: PMC8757760.

53. Okamura AM, Simone C, O'leary MD. Force modeling for needle insertion into soft tissue. *IEEE Trans Biomed Eng.* 2004;51(10):1707–1716. doi:10.1109/tbme.2004.831542.

54. Pradhan B, Bharti D, Chakravarty S, Ray SS, Voinova VV, Bonartsev AP, et al. Internet of things and robotics in transforming current-day healthcare services. *J Healthc Eng.* 2021 May 26;2021:9999504. doi:10.1155/2021/9999504. PMID: 34104368; PMCID: PMC8158416.

55. Gatouillat A, Badr Y, Massot B, Sejdic E. Internet of medical things: a review of recent contributions dealing with cyber-physical systems in medicine. *IEEE Internet Things J.* 2018;5(5):3810–3822. doi:10.1109/jiot.2018.2849014.

56. Nasiri S, Sadoughi F, Tadayon MH, Dehnad A. Security requirements of internet of things-based healthcare system: a survey study. *Acta Inform Med.* 2019 Dec;27(4):253–258. doi:10.5455/aim.2019.27.253-258. PMID: 32055092; PMCID: PMC7004290.

57. Calabrò RS, Cacciola A, Bertè F, Manuli A, Leo A, Bramanti A, et al. Robotic gait rehabilitation and substitution devices in neurological disorders: where are we now? *Neurol Sci.* 2016;37(4):503–514.

58. Bertani R, Melegari C, De Cola MC, Bramanti A, Bramanti P, Calabrò RS. Effects of robot-assisted upper limb rehabilitation in stroke patients: a systematic review with meta-analysis. *Neurol Sci.* 2017;38(9):1561–1569.

59. Dobkin BH. Strategies for stroke rehabilitation. *Lancet Neurol.* 2004 Sep;3(9):528–536. doi:10.1016/S1474-4422(04)00851-8. PMID: 15324721; PMCID: PMC4164204.

60. Morgan AA, Abdi J, Syed MAQ, Kohen GE, Barlow P, Vizcaychipi MP. Robots in healthcare: a scoping review. *Curr Robot Rep.* 2022;3(4): 271–280. doi:10.1007/s43154-022-00095-4. Epub 2022 Oct 22. PMID: 36311256; PMCID: PMC9589563.

61. Sultan N. Reflective thoughts on the potential and challenges of wearable technology for healthcare provision and medical education. *Int J Inf Manag.* 2015;35:521–526. doi:10.1016/j.ijinfomgt.2015.04.010.

62. Chen TL, Ciocarlie M, Cousins S, Grice PM, Hawkins K, Hsiao K, et al. Robots for humanity: using assistive robotics to empower people with disabilities. *IEEE Robot Autom Mag.* 2013;20:30–39. doi:10.1109/MRA.2012.2229950.

63. Chen B, Ma H, Qin LY, Gao F, Chan KM, Law SW, et al. Recent developments and challenges of lower extremity exoskeletons. *J Orthop Transl.* 2016;5:26–37. doi:10.1016/j.jot.2015.09.007.

64. Esquenazi A, Talaty M, Packel A, Saulino M. The ReWalk powered exoskeleton to restore ambulatory function to individuals with thoracic-level motor-complete spinal cord injury. *Am J Phys Med Rehabil.* 2012 Nov;91(11):911–921. doi:10.1097/PHM.0b013e318269d9a3. PMID: 23085703.

65. Matarić MJ, Eriksson J, Feil-Seifer DJ, Winstein CJ. Socially assistive robotics for post-stroke rehabilitation. *J NeuroEng Rehabil.* 2007;4:5. doi:10.1186/1743-0003-4-5.

66. Akbari A, Haghverd F, Behbahani S. Robotic home-based rehabilitation systems design: from a literature review to a conceptual framework for community-based remote therapy during COVID-19 pandemic. *Front Robot AI.* 2021 Jun 22;8:612331. doi:10.3389/frobt.2021.612331. PMID: 34239898; PMCID: PMC8258116.

67. Volpe BT, Krebs HI, Hogan N. Is robot-aided sensorimotor training in stroke rehabilitation a realistic option? *Curr Opin Neurol.* 2001;14(6): 745–752.

68. Kaelin VC, Valizadeh M, Salgado Z, Parde N, Khetani MA. Artificial intelligence in rehabilitation targeting the participation of children and youth

with disabilities: scoping review. *J Med Internet Res.* 2021;23:e25745. doi:10.2196/25745.

69. Gorgey A, Sumrell R, Goetz L. Exoskeletal assisted rehabilitation after spinal cord injury. In: Webster JB, Murphy DP, editor. *Atlas of Orthoses and Assistive Devices.* 5th ed. Canada: Elsevier; 2018. p. 440–447.

70. Gorgey AS. Robotic exoskeletons: the current pros and cons. *World J Orthop.* 2018 Sep 18;9(9):112–119. doi:10.5312/wjo.v9.i9.112. PMID: 30254967; PMCID: PMC6153133.

71. Ai QS, Liu ZM, Meng W, Liu Q, Xie SQ.Machine learning in robot-assisted upper limb rehabilitation: a focused review. *IEEE Trans Cogn Dev Syst.* 2023;15(4). https://doi.org/10.1109/TCDS.2021.3098350.

72. Kristoffersson A, Coradeschi S, Loutfi A. A review of mobile robotic telepresence. *Adv Hum Computer Interact.* 2013;2013:17. Article ID 902316. doi:10.1155/2013/902316.

73. Surgical Telepresence Technology Connects Remote Areas to World-Class Healthcare. Med Journal 360. https://mcdjournal360.com/internal-medicine/surgical-telepresence-technology-connects-remote-areas-to-world-class-healthcare/. Accessed 2023 Dec 18.

74. Maibaum A, Bischof A, Hergesell J, Lipp B. A critique of robotics in health care. *AI Soc.* 2021;37:467–477. doi:10.1007/s00146-021-01206-z.

75. Petelin JB, Nelson ME, Goodman J. Deployment and early experience with remote-presence patient care in a community hospital. *Surg Endosc Other Interv Tech.* 2007;21(1):53–56.

76. Bemelmans R, Gelderblom GJ, Jonker P, de Witte L. Socially assistive robots in elderly care: a systematic review into effects and effectiveness. *J Am Med Dir Assoc.* 2012 Feb;13(2):114–120.e1. doi:10.1016/j.jamda. 2010.10.002. Epub 2010 Dec 15. PMID: 21450215.

77. Hung L, Wong J, Smith C, Berndt A, Gregorio M, Horne N, et al. Facilitators and barriers to using telepresence robots in aged care settings: a scoping review. *J Rehabil Assist Technol Eng.* 2022;21:9. doi: 10.1177/20556683211072385.

78. McCann E. RP-VITA Robot Promises to Reboot Healthcare. Healthcare IT News; 2012. https://www.healthcareitnews.com/news/rp-vita-robot-promises-reboot-healthcare. Accessed 2023 Dec 12.

79. OhmniLabs. *Exploring Telepresence Technology — A Guide to Boundless Communication.* 2023. https://ohmnilabs.com/telepresence/exploring-telepresence-technology-a-guide-to-boundless-communication/. Accessed 2023 Dec 18.

80. Raison N, Khan MS, Challacombe B. Telemedicine in surgery: what are the opportunities and hurdles to realising the potential? *Curr Urol Rep.* 2015;16:43.

81. Satava RM. Surgical robotics: the early chronicles: a personal historical perspective. *Surg Laparosc Endosc Percutaneous Tech.* 2012;12:6–16.

82. Marescaux J, Leroy J, Gagner M, Mutter D, Vix M, Butner SE, et al. Transatlantic robot-assisted telesurgery. *Nature.* 2001;413:379–380. doi:10.1038/35096636.

83. PillPick® Automated Packaging and Dispensing System. Swisslog Healthcare. 2024. https://www.swisslog-healthcare.com/en-us/products/pharmacy-automation/pillpick-automated-packaging-and-dispensing-system. Accessed 2023 Dec 12.

84. Tu HN, Shan TH, Wu YC, Shen PH, Wu TY, Lin WL, et al. Reducing medication errors by adopting automatic dispensing cabinets in critical care units. *J Med Syst.* 2023 Apr 27;47(1):52. doi:10.1007/s10916-023-01953-0. PMID: 37103718; PMCID: PMC10136387.

85. Jiménez Muñoz AB, Muiño Miguez A, Rodriguez Pérez MP, Garcia MED, Saez MS. Comparison of medication error rates and clinical effects in three medication prescription-dispensation systems. *Int J Health Care Qual Assur.* 2011;24:238–248.

86. Takase T, Masumoto N, Shibatani N, Matsuoka Y, Tanaka F, Hirabatake M, et al. Evaluating the safety and efficiency of robotic dispensing systems. *J Pharm Health Care Sci.* 2022 Oct 1;8(1):24. doi:10.1186/s40780-022-00255-w. PMID: 36180937; PMCID: PMC9526262.

87. Momattin H, Arafa S, Momattin S, Rahal R, Waterson J. Robotic pharmacy implementation and outcomes in Saudi Arabia: a 21-Month usability study. *JMIR Hum Factors.* 2021 Sep 1;8(3):e28381. doi:10.2196/28381. PMID: 34304149; PMCID: PMC8444036.

88. How Robots Are Redefining Health Care: 6 Recent Innovations. Robotics Tomorrow. 2024. https://www.roboticstomorrow.com/story/2022/03/how-robots-are-redefining-health-care-6-recent-innovations/18339/. Accessed 2023 Jan 2.

89. Ramos CCR, Roque JLA, Sarmiento DB, Suarez LEG, Sunio JTP, Tabungar KIB, et al. Use of ultraviolet-C in environmental sterilization in hospitals: a systematic review on efficacy and safety. *Int J Health Sci (Qassim).* 2020 Nov-Dec;14(6):52–65. PMID: 33192232; PMCID: PMC7644456.

90. Javaid M, Haleem A, Singh RP, Rab S, Suman R, Kumar L. Utilization of robotics for healthcare: a scoping review. *J Ind Integr Manag.* 2022;7:1–23. doi:10.1142/S2424862222500154.

91. Mumtaz H, Saqib M, Jabeen S, Muneeb M, Mughal W, Sohai H, et al. Exploring alternative approaches to precision medicine through genomics and artificial intelligence — a systematic review. *Front Med.* 2023;10: 1227168. doi:10.3389/fmed.2023.1227168.

92. Intuitive. *Exploring New Advancements in Robotics.* 2024. https://www. intuitive.com/en-us/about-us/newsroom/exploring-new-advancements-in-robotics. Accessed 2023 Dec 30.

93. Intuitive. *Intuitive's Sophisticated Digital Tools help Bring Robotic Surgery to the Next Level.* 2024. https://www.intuitive.com/en-us/about-us/news-room/integrated-intelligence. Accessed 12/30/23.

94. Hassabis D. *AlphaGo: Using Machine Learning to Master the Ancient Game of Go.* 2016. https://blog.google/technology/ai/alphago-machine-learning-game-go/. Accessed 2023 Dec 30.

95. Hashimoto DA, Rosman G, Rus D, Meireles OR. Artificial intelligence in surgery: promises and perils. *Ann Surg.* 2018 Jul;268(1):70–76. doi:10.1097/ SLA.0000000000002693. PMID: 29389679; PMCID: PMC5995666.

96. Alaska Airlines. 2021. https://news.alaskaair.com/newsroom/alaska-airlines-and-airspace-intelligence-announce-first-of-its-kind-partnership-to-optimize-air-traffic-flow-with-artificial-intelligence-and-machine-learning/#:~:text=Flyways%20AI%20is%20a%204D,airline's%20 planned%20and%20active%20flights. Accessed 2023 Dec 30.

97. Satapathy P, Hermis AH, Rustagi S, Pradhan KB, Padhi BK, Sah R. Artificial intelligence in surgical education and training: opportunities, challenges, and ethical considerations - correspondence. *Int J Surg.* 2023 May 1;109(5):1543–1544. doi:10.1097/JS9.0000000000000387. PMID: 37037597; PMCID: PMC10389387.

98. Rogers MP, DeSantis AJ, Janjua H, Barry TM, Kuo PC. The future surgical training paradigm: virtual reality and machine learning in surgical educa-tion. *Surg (US).* 2021;169(5):1250–1252.

99. Rubalcava NS, Guetter CR, Kapani N, Quiñones PM. *How Artificial Intelligence Is Expected to Transform Surgical Training.* Chicago: American College of Surgeons; 2023. https://www.facs.org/for-medical-professionals/ news-publications/news-and-articles/bulletin/2023/august-2023-volume-108-issue-8/how-artificial-intelligence-is-expected-to-transform-surgical-training/. Accessed 2023 Dec 30.

100. Hettiarachchi TS, Askari A, Rudge E, Hao LT, Sarwar S, Dowsett D, et al. Comparison of robotic vs laparoscopic left-sided colorectal cancer resections. *J Robotic Surg.* 2023;17:205–213. doi:10.1007/s11701-022-01414-9.

101. Garg H, Psutka SP, Hakimi AA, Kim HL, Mansour AM, Pruthi DK, et al. A decade of robotic-assisted radical nephrectomy with inferior vena cava thrombectomy: a systematic review and meta-analysis of perioperative outcomes. *J Urol.* 2022 Sep1;208:542–560. doi:10.1097/ JU.0000000000002829.

102. Wang Y, Cao D, Chen SL, Li YM, Zheng YW, Ohkohchi N. Current trends in three-dimensional visualization and real-time navigation as well as robot-assisted technologies in hepatobiliary surgery. *World J Gastrointest Surg.* 2021;13:904–922. doi:10.4240/wjgs.v13.i9.904.

103. Troy Miner. Improving healthcare accessibility with robotics. Ziva ROBOTICS. 2023. https://www.zivarobotics.com/robotics-in-healthcare-accessibility/#:~:text=However%2C%20challenges%20such%20as%20 the,will%20further%20revolutionize%20patient%20care. Accessed 2024 Jan 1.

104. Qureshi MO, Syed RS. The impact of robotics on employment and motiva-tion of employees in the service sector, with special reference to health care. *Saf Health Work.* 2014 Dec;5(4):198–202. doi:10.1016/j.shaw.2014.07.003. Epub 2014 Jul 29. PMID: 25516812; PMCID: PMC4266810.

105. Abdel Raheem A, Song HJ, Chang KD, Choi YD, Rha KH. Robotic nurse duties in the urology operative room: 11 years of experience. *Asian J Urol.* 2017 Apr;4(2):116–123. doi:10.1016/j.ajur.2016.09.012. Epub 2017 Jan 20. PMID: 29264216; PMCID: PMC5717981.

106. Tietze M, Mcbride S. *Robotics and the Impact on Nursing Practice.* Maryland: American Nurse Association. chrome-extension://efaidn-bmnnnibpcajpcglclefindmkaj/https://www.nursingworld.org/~494055/ globalassets/innovation/robotics-and-the-impact-on-nursing-practice_ print_12-2-2020-pdf-1.pdf. Accessed 2024 Jan 2.

107. Dias J, Khanna S, Paquette C, Rohr M, Seitz B, Singla A, et al. *Introducing the Next-Generation Operating Model.* New York: McKinsey & Company; 2017. chrome-extension://efaidnbmnnnibpcajpcglclefindmkaj/https://www. mckinsey.com/~/media/mckinsey/business%20functions/mckinsey%20 digital/our%20insights/introducing%20the%20next-generation%20operat-ing%20model/introducing-the-next-gen-operating-model.ashx. Accessed 2024 Jan 2.

108. Fosch-Villaronga E, Khanna P, Drukarch H, Custers B. The role of humans in surgery automation. *Int J of Soc Robotics.* 2023;15:563–580. doi:10.1007/ s12369-022-00875-0.

109. Green CA, Mahuron KM, Harris HW, O''Sullivan PS. Integrating robotic technology into resident training: challenges and recommendations from the front lines. *Acad Med.* 2019 Oct;94(10):1532–1538. doi:10.1097/ACM.0000000000002751. PMID: 30998574; PMCID: PMC6768698.

110. Mlambo M, Silén C, McGrath C. Lifelong learning and nurses' continuing professional development, a metasynthesis of the literature. *BMC Nurs.* 2021;20:62. doi:10.1186/s12912-021-00579-2.

111. Soriano GP, Yasuhara Y, Ito H, Matsumoto K, Osaka K, Kai Y, et al. Robots and robotics in nursing. *Healthcare (Basel).* 2022 Aug 18; 10(8):1571. doi:10.3390/healthcare10081571. PMID: 36011228; PMCID: PMC9407759.

112. Weerarathna IN, Raymond D, Luharia A. Human-robot collaboration for healthcare: a narrative review. *Cureus.* 2023 Nov 21;15(11):e49210. doi:10.7759/cureus.49210. PMID: 38143700; PMCID: PMC10739095.

113. *Roboticists' Role in Healthcare and Medicine.* Evanston: Northwestern University; 2022. https://www.mccormick.northwestern.edu/robotics/inside-our-program/stories/2022/roboticists-role-in-healthcare-and-medicine.html. Accessed 2024 Jan 4.

114. Holzer HJ. *Understanding the Impact of Automation on Workers, Jobs, and Wages.* Washington, DC: The Brookings Institution; 2022. https://www.brookings.edu/articles/understanding-the-impact-of-automation-on-workers-jobs-and-wages/. Accessed 2024 Jan 4.

115. Maynou L, McGuire A, Serra-Sastre V. Efficiency and productivity gains of robotic surgery: the case of the English National Health Service. SSRN: https://ssrn.com/abstract=4305820. doi:10.2139/ssrn.4305820.

116. Smith A, Anderson J. *AI, Robotics, and the Future of Jobs.* Washington, DC: Pew Research Center; 2014. https://www.pewresearch.org/internet/2014/08/06/future-of-jobs/. Accessed 2024 Jan 4.

117. Acemoglu D, Restrepo P. Automation and new tasks: how technology displaces and reinstates labor. *J Econ Perspect.* 2019;33(2):3–30.

118. Sharkey A, Sharkey N. Granny and the robots: ethical issues in robot care for the elderly. *Ethics and Inf. Technol.* 2012 Mar;14(1):27–40. doi:10.1007/s10676-010-9234-6.

119. Broekens J, Heerink M, Rosendal H. Assistive social robots in elderly care: a review. *Gerontechnology.* 2009;8(2):94–103.

120. Turkle S. *Alone Together: Why We Expect More from Technology and Less from Each Other.* 3rd ed. New York: Basic Books; 2017 Nov 7.

Chapter 4

Beyond the Clinic: Wearable Monitors and mHealth Apps Transforming Healthcare

Introduction

In the evolving landscape of digital health, two pivotal technologies have emerged as key players in transforming patient care and health management: wearable monitors and mobile health (mHealth) applications. These devices represent two distinct approaches in digital health technology, each with its unique mode of operation and patient interaction.

This chapter focuses on the burgeoning field of mobile digital monitoring and its role in enhancing patient engagement, shared decision-making, and self-management in healthcare. We delve into the various categories of devices and apps related to care coordination, medication management, and chronic disease management, emphasizing clinically validated and user-friendly options for patients.

We will explore these innovative tools, examining their functionalities, benefits, and roles in modern healthcare.

Wearable Monitors

Wearable monitors, a subset of digital health technologies, are devices designed to be worn on the body and used by patients outside of traditional healthcare settings. They can take the form of smartwatches, smart rings, and adhesive patches with sensors, to name a few.

Wearable devices ingeniously combine mechanical functions with microelectronics and computing capabilities. This integration enables them to promptly detect patient signs and laboratory indicators. They can offer a range of services, including exercise guidance and reminders for medication administration. The primary goal of these devices is to facilitate multiparameter, real-time, and online monitoring. They provide accurate and intelligent analysis of human physiological and pathological information. This advanced functionality allows individuals to self-diagnose and self-monitor, enhancing personal health management.[1]

These tools automatically collect and analyze activity levels and physiological data, offering real-time insights into an individual's health status. They are designed to passively collect health data, requiring minimal to no active input from the patient in contrast to the mHealth apps that require the patient to input the data. Their defining feature is their ability to provide ongoing health monitoring in a nonintrusive, user-friendly manner, making them invaluable for preventive health measures and managing chronic conditions.

The following are the critical characteristics of wearable monitors:

- Portability: They are designed to be easily carried or worn by the patient, facilitating mobility and use in various environments, including at home, work, or on the go.
- Connectivity: Many of these devices can connect to smartphones, tablets, or computers, allowing data transmission to healthcare providers or patients to view and manage their health information.
- Functionality: They serve various medical purposes, from monitoring vital signs (such as blood pressure monitors and pulse oximeters) to providing therapeutic interventions (such as portable insulin pumps).
- User-Friendly Design: They are generally designed for ease of use by patients, often featuring intuitive interfaces and clear instructions.
- Regulatory Oversight: Depending on their intended use and risk level, mobile medical devices may be subject to regulatory oversight to ensure their safety and efficacy.

They can range from simple, manually operated tools to sophisticated devices integrated with software, sensors, and wireless communication capabilities. The following are some examples of these devices:

- Fitness Trackers: Devices such as the Fitbit or Apple Watch automatically track heart rate, steps, and sometimes even blood oxygen levels throughout the day.
- Continuous Glucose Monitors (CGMs): Devices such as the Dexcom G6 attach to the body and continuously monitor glucose levels, sending data to a smartphone or a receiver.[2]
- Wearable Electrocardiogram (ECG) Monitors: Devices such as the Zio Patch are worn on the chest and continuously record heart activity. They are often used to diagnose arrhythmias.[3]

The market for these devices is growing significantly. By 2022, more than a million smart rings will have been sold, and more than 7 million CGMs will be sold in 2023.[4] Bloomberg predicts that the wearables market will exceed $76 billion by 2028.[5]

In the realm of wearable monitors, there are several categories, each serving different health needs. Fitness and activity trackers, such as Fitbit and Garmin watches, are primarily focused on tracking physical activities, heart rate, and sleep patterns, making them ideal for individuals keen on maintaining a healthy lifestyle or monitoring basic health metrics. Advanced health monitors, such as the Apple Watch, offer more than just fitness tracking; they include features such as ECG monitoring and fall detection, which are particularly beneficial for patients with cardiac conditions or elderly individuals.

Specialized medical wearables are another category, encompassing devices such as the Holter monitor, CGMs such as the Dexcom G6, and blood pressure monitoring devices. These are specifically designed for patients with medical conditions such as heart arrhythmias, diabetes, or hypertension that require close monitoring. Wearable biosensors represent the more advanced end of the spectrum, capable of measuring diverse physiological data, including skin temperature, sweat analysis, and oxygen saturation. These are typically used in clinical research and for specialized care.

The impact of wearable mobile medical devices on diagnoses and patient outcomes is profound. For example, wearable devices significantly enhance patient engagement by providing real-time health and fitness data, encouraging patients to participate in their care actively.[6] This leads to better adherence to treatment plans and fosters positive lifestyle changes. For example, a heart rate monitor can help patients manage their cardiovascular health more proactively, or a continuous EKG monitor can identify irregular heart rhythms, enabling timely medical intervention.

In remote monitoring, healthcare professionals can keep track of patients' vital signs and health metrics from a distance. Monitoring vital signs is an aid in detecting clinical deterioration, and changes in these parameters may occur several hours before an adverse event.[7,8] This is especially beneficial for individuals with chronic conditions[9] or those recovering from surgery, as it allows for informed decisions and timely interventions when necessary.[10] For instance, a wearable device that monitors blood glucose levels can be crucial for a diabetic patient's ongoing care. They can play an essential role in maintaining better glycemic control, thereby reducing the risk of complications.

Wearable technology also plays a pivotal role in enhancing research and treatment monitoring.[11] It enables tracking treatment effectiveness, medication adherence, and patient experiences, leading to more comprehensive and accurate research outcomes. For example, data from wearable blood pressure monitors used by participants can enhance a study on the effectiveness of a new hypertension drug.

Additionally, wearable technology contributes to reducing healthcare costs. Allowing individuals to monitor their vital signs and health in real time reduces the need for expensive hospital visits and unnecessary medical treatments.[12,13] This leads to more efficient and effective medical care, ultimately cutting healthcare expenses. For example, a 2021 study in *Nature* revealed that using wearable devices for remote monitoring significantly reduced hospital readmissions by 43% among patients with type I myocardial infarction (MI), a coronary artery disease.[14] Through continuous fitness monitoring and timely health interventions, these devices helped prevent complications and reduced hospitalization needs, saving an average of $6,000 per patient.

Lastly, data-driven decisions are a significant advantage of wearable technology. It provides healthcare professionals and patients with insights based on extensive information about a person's health and activity levels gathered through wearable devices. This abundance of data supports informed decision-making, enhancing the overall quality of healthcare. For example, a fitness tracker's data can help a physician tailor an exercise program to a patient's health needs.

mHealth Apps: Definition and Scope

The widespread accessibility of the smartphone in the past two decades has changed how people monitor their health.[15,16] Indeed, as of 2018, 95% of U.S. adults own a cell phone,[17,18] and they carry these phones on them most of the day. They are making[19] the cell phone a convenient and accessible device for health management *on the go*.[20] In addition, more than 84 million people in the United States use apps with health and health-related content.

The U.S. Food and Drug Administration (FDA) defines mHealth apps, short for mobile health applications, as mobile software that diagnoses, tracks, or treats disease.[21] These software programs are developed for mobile devices such as smartphones, tablets, or watches,[22] and they can promote patient health and aid in disease prevention.[23] They can also help increase patient autonomy[24] and treatment adherence[25] while decreasing medical costs.[26]

These devices typically involve more active patient participation than digital health monitors. They require the patient to manually input health data or perform a specific action to gather health information.

The scope of these apps is broad and varied. They can range from simple tools that provide users with medical information and advice to more complex systems capable of tracking and monitoring vital signs such as heart rate[27] and blood pressure.[28] Some mHealth apps are designed to assist in managing specific health conditions, such as diabetes, by helping users monitor their blood sugar levels and medication schedules.[29] Others might be focused on mental health, offering resources for stress management, mindfulness, or therapy support.[30]

Additionally, mHealth apps facilitate telemedicine, allowing patients to consult with healthcare professionals remotely. Examples of mHealth apps include MyFitnessPal,[31] a nutrition and exercise tracker; Headspace,[32] for mindfulness and meditation; and Teladoc,[33] which provides access to medical consultations via video calls.

Currently, these apps are only loosely regulated, and laws specific to apps are rare.

Wearable Monitor Versus mHealth App

The primary difference between wearable monitors and mHealth apps lies in the required level of patient engagement. mHealth apps require active patient input and are generally used for specific, periodic health measurements. In contrast, wearable medical monitors are more about passive data collection, providing continuous monitoring without active patient involvement. This difference in patient engagement can influence the choice of a device based on the patient's condition, lifestyle, and preference for interaction with their health monitoring tools.

Evolution and Rapid Growth of mHealth in Patient Care

The mHealth market has seen exponential growth, driven by the widespread adoption of smartphones and advancements in digital health technology. This growth transforms how patients and healthcare providers interact and manage health and wellness.[34]

The Potential of mHealth in Transforming Healthcare Delivery

mHealth apps can significantly improve healthcare delivery by enhancing access to care, personalizing treatment, and reducing healthcare costs.[35]

Categories of mHealth Apps

Care Coordination Apps

Apps that focus on facilitating communication and coordination play a crucial role in healthcare by strengthening the continuity of care and minimizing the likelihood of errors. These applications serve as a bridge between healthcare providers and patients, ensuring that all parties are consistently informed and aligned in understanding the patient's care plan.[36] By providing a platform for seamless information exchange, these apps help maintain an ongoing, coherent treatment process, even when multiple providers are involved.[37] This continuous flow of information can significantly reduce misunderstandings or information gaps that might lead to errors in patient care. Examples include apps such as Cerner's CareAware or Epic's MyChart, which have been instrumental in streamlining patient–provider communication and improving care coordination.

Medication Management Apps

Medication management applications are designed to assist patients in engaging with their treatment plans and effectively managing their medication regimens.[38] Increasing engagement in their treatment improves a patient's compliance with their treatment.[39] Mobile apps can offer patients tools to enhance their engagement in the treatment and well-being.[40,41] The apps achieve this by providing features such as reminders for when to take medications, tracking systems for dosages, and tools to monitor adherence to prescribed treatment plans. Some apps allow the patient to monitor and track health parameters related to the medication (e.g., blood glucose level, HbA1c, and weight). Others can alert users about the need for a prescription renewal. In their study, Ahmed et al. explored various strategies to improve adherence through apps, including gamification elements and typical reminder functions.[25]

These functionalities are vital in ensuring patients follow their medication schedules accurately, which is essential for optimal treatment outcomes.[42] Examples of such apps include Medisafe,[43] which provides personalized reminders and a medication tracker, and MyTherapy,[44] known for its pill reminder and health journal features.

These apps have been shown to improve adherence rates and patient outcomes by providing reminders and tracking capabilities.[45,46]

Chronic Disease Management Apps

Apps designed for managing chronic conditions such as diabetes, hypertension, and asthma are increasingly becoming integral to patient care. The goal of mHealth apps is to increase self-management of chronic diseases, which plays a central role in improving clinical outcomes.[47,48] These apps typically include features for monitoring various health parameters relevant to the specific condition. For instance, diabetes management apps may have functionalities for tracking blood glucose levels, carbohydrate intake, and insulin doses.[49] Hypertension apps might focus on monitoring blood pressure and heart rate, while asthma apps could include symptom diaries and peak flow meter recordings.

These apps often incorporate medication adherence tools, such as reminders for taking medication at prescribed times, which is crucial for conditions requiring strict medication regimens. By providing these reminders and enabling patients to log their medication intake, these apps help ensure that patients follow their treatment plans more closely, reducing the likelihood of complications associated with nonadherence.

Furthermore, many of these apps engage patients more actively in their health management by offering educational content, personalized feedback, and interactive features. This increased engagement can lead to better self-management of the condition, fostering a sense of control and empowerment among patients.[50]

Improved patient outcomes are a significant benefit of these apps. By enabling better disease monitoring, enhancing medication adherence, and increasing patient engagement, these apps can contribute to better disease control, reduced hospitalizations, and overall improved quality of life for patients with chronic conditions.[51,52]

Examples of such apps include MySugr, a diabetes management app that specializes in logging blood sugar levels, insulin use, and carbohydrate intake; OMRON Connect, a blood pressure monitoring app that works with compatible Omron blood pressure cuffs; and AsthmaMD, an app that allows asthma patients to track their symptoms, medication usage, and peak flow readings.

Benefits of mHealth Apps for Patient Engagement and Shared Decision-Making

Enhanced Patient Engagement

Research indicates that higher levels of patient engagement are associated with better health outcomes and more efficient healthcare utilization.[53] mHealth apps foster active patient participation in their healthcare, leading to increased engagement. These apps offer a variety of tools and resources that empower patients to take a more active role in managing their health.

One crucial way these apps encourage active participation is through personalized health tracking. Many apps allow patients to monitor vital health metrics relevant to their conditions, such as blood glucose levels in diabetes, blood pressure in hypertension, or symptom patterns in chronic illnesses such as asthma. This ensures better management of their condition and educates them about their medication, fostering a deeper understanding of their treatment.

Additionally, many mHealth apps include educational content tailored to the user's health conditions. This information helps patients better understand their health, informing them about their conditions and treatments. Apps such as WebMD[54] offer a wealth of information on various health topics, enabling patients to educate themselves beyond the doctor's office.

Interactive features such as symptom checkers, virtual consultations, and health challenges significantly increase engagement. For instance, the Symptomate[55] app uses an AI-driven symptom checker to help users identify potential health issues and seek appropriate care.

Furthermore, some apps use gamification to encourage healthy behaviors. For example, MyFitnessPal[31] incorporates gamified elements to motivate users to achieve their diet and exercise goals, making the process more engaging and enjoyable.

How mHealth Apps Support Informed and Collaborative Decision-Making

Shared decision-making is defined as "an approach where clinicians and patients share the best available evidence when faced with the task of making decisions, and where patients are supported to consider options, to achieve informed preferences."[56] Shared decision-making is necessary to support the ethical tenets of patient self-determination[57] and autonomy.[58] mHealth apps provide patients access to their health information, enabling informed discussions and shared decision-making with healthcare providers.[59] Evidence suggests that shared decision-making leads to higher patient satisfaction and adherence to treatment plans.[60–62]

Ensuring Clinical Validity

To ensure their safety and effectiveness, mHealth apps must be based on scientific evidence and clinical validation. Healthcare providers should assess apps based on their development process, clinical evidence, regulatory approval, and user reviews. By thoroughly evaluating these aspects, healthcare providers can recommend mHealth apps to their patients, ensuring that these digital tools are effective and safe and align with their patient's specific needs and circumstances.

User-Friendly Design

The design of mHealth apps should prioritize ease of use, accessibility, and engagement to ensure they are effective for a diverse range of users.[63] Factors to consider include readability, navigation ease, language options, and the inclusion of assistive technologies for users with disabilities. The effectiveness of mHealth apps is heavily influenced by their user experience and interface design. These aspects are crucial because they directly impact how easily and effectively users interact with the app, affecting their willingness to use it and adhere to its recommendations or features.

Ease of use is a critical factor in mHealth app design. If an app is complicated or unintuitive, users, especially those who may be less tech-savvy or have limited experience with digital technology, might find it challenging to use. This difficulty can lead to frustration, decreased engagement, and, ultimately, abandonment of the app. For instance, older adults or individuals with specific disabilities might struggle with small text sizes or complex navigation menus. Therefore, designing apps with simple, straightforward interfaces and providing options such as adjustable text sizes can significantly improve accessibility and usability for these groups.

Accessibility is another critical aspect. This includes making the app usable for people with disabilities (such as incorporating screen reader compatibility for visually impaired users) and ensuring the app can be used across various devices and platforms. This broad accessibility ensures that a more comprehensive range of users can benefit from the app, regardless of their device type or physical limitations.

Engagement is also closely tied to design. A visually appealing app that provides personalized feedback and includes interactive elements are more likely to keep users engaged. Gamification elements, for example, can make tracking health metrics or adhering to treatment more engaging and less monotonous. Apps such as MyFitnessPal use these techniques to encourage users to log their food intake and exercise regularly.

What Type of Device Should a Patient Get?

Determining the suitability of a wearable mobile monitor versus a mHealth app for a patient involves considering their specific health needs, lifestyle, comfort with technology, and the extent of monitoring or interaction their condition necessitates.

Wearable mobile monitors are particularly beneficial for patients with chronic conditions such as diabetes, heart disease, or hypertension. These devices, such as CGMs for diabetics or heart rate monitors for cardiac patients, provide essential real-time data for managing these conditions. They are also ideal for conditions that require constant vigilance, such as arrhythmias or sleep apnea, offering continuous, real-time monitoring. Elderly patients, especially those at risk of falls or sudden health changes, can benefit significantly from wearables equipped with fall detection and emergency alert systems. Additionally, wearables are advantageous for patients in physical rehabilitation, tracking movement patterns, progress, and physical activity levels.

On the other hand, mHealth apps are well suited for individuals focusing on general health and wellness, such as fitness tracking, diet monitoring, and mental well-being. They are also appropriate for managing conditions that do not demand constant monitoring, such as mild asthma or occasional migraines. Tech-savvy patients who are comfortable using smartphones and prefer digital healthcare management, including appointments and prescriptions, may find mHealth apps more user-friendly. Moreover, these apps are valuable for patients seeking educational resources about their conditions, treatments, and health maintenance strategies.

Often, a combination of both wearable monitors and mHealth apps can provide a comprehensive approach, particularly for patients with complex health needs. Wearables can supply the necessary continuous monitoring data, while mHealth apps can enhance this with medication reminders, educational content, and a platform for healthcare provider communication.

This approach to determining the most suitable digital health tool considers patients' diverse needs and preferences, ensuring that the chosen technology aligns well with their specific healthcare requirements.

Conclusion

The healthcare landscape is being profoundly reshaped by the advent of wearable medical devices and mHealth apps. These technologies bridge the gap between traditional healthcare settings and patients' daily lives, offering unprecedented opportunities for continuous health monitoring, enhanced patient engagement, and more personalized care. Wearable devices provide vital insights into a patient's health status, facilitating early detection of potential issues and more effective management of chronic conditions. Simultaneously, mHealth apps empower patients with tools to better manage their health, from medication adherence to accessing medical information and support. Together, these innovations are transforming how healthcare is delivered and experienced, paving the way for a more proactive, patient-centered, and data-driven approach to health and wellness. As we continue to embrace and integrate these technologies, their potential to improve healthcare outcomes, reduce costs, and enhance the quality of life for patients worldwide becomes increasingly evident.

References

1. Guk K, Han G, Lim J, Jeong K, Kang T, Lim E et al. Evolution of wearable devices with real-time disease monitoring for personalized health care. *Nanomaterials (Basel).* 2019 May 29;9(6):813. doi:10.3390/nano9060813. https://www.mdpi.com/resolver?pii=nano9060813.
2. Dexcom. https://www.dexcom.com/get-started-cgm/203?sfc=7014y000001e D4kAAE&gad_source=1&gclid=Cj0KCQiAtOmsBhCnARIsAGPa5ybRnO 9HGfgjIpeK-PV0YelSKPjSL3jWGvN_CtY0VuGkhtywOVzx FtoaAuGgEALw_wcB&gclsrc=aw.ds. Accessed 2024 Jan 7.
3. Zio. https://www.irhythmtech.com/providers/zio-service/zio-monitors. Accessed 2024 Jan 7.
4. Stephen HF, Geoffrey SG, Rosalind WP. Wearable digital health technology. *N Engl J Med.* 2023;389:2100–2101. doi:10.1056/NEJMe2303219.
5. Bloomberg. *Wearable Medical Devices Market to Grow US$ 76,479.8 mn by end of 2028, Says Coherent Market Insights.* New York: Bloomberg; 2021 Oct 20. https://www.bloomberg.com/press-releases/2021-10-20/wearable-medical-devices-market-to-grow-us-76-479-8-mn-by-end-of-2028-says-coherent-market-insights. opens in new tab. Accessed 2024 Jan 7.
6. Stronghold Data. The Role of Wearable Technology in Healthcare. Stronghold Data. 2023. https://strongholddata.com/wearable-technology-in-healthcare/. Accessed 2024 Jan 8.
7. DeVita MA, Smith GB, Adam SK, Adams-Pizarro I, Buist M, Bellomo R, et al. "Identifying the hospitalised patient in crisis" — a consensus conference on the afferent limb of rapid response systems. *Resuscitation.* 2010;81:375–382.
8. Smith GB. In-hospital cardiac arrest: is it time for an in-hospital 'chain of prevention'? *Resuscitation.* 2010;81:1209–1211.

9. The Future of Healthcare: How Wearable Devices Are Transforming Patient Care. Wearable Devices. 2023. https://www.linkedin.com/pulse/future-healthcare-how-wearable-devices-transforming-patient-care/. Accessed 2024 Jan 8.

10. Prajapati N. Wearable Technology: An Emerging Future Trend in mHealth. Syndell. 2023. https://syndelltech.com/wearables-an-emerging-future-trend-in-mhealth-apps/. Accessed 2024 Jan 8.

11. mSafety for Clinical Trials. Sony. https://www.sonynetworkcom.com/msafety/clinicaltrials?utm_campaign=C25102023-mSafety-GAds-Search-Traffic-Pharma-FY23&utm_source=ppc&utm_source=adwords&utm_medium=ppc&utm_campaign=C10102023-mSafety-Search-Ads-Pharma-FY23&utm_term=wearables%20in%20clinical%20trials&hsa_net=adwords&hsa_kw=wearables%20in%20clinical%20trials&hsa_mt=b&hsa_cam=20701305801&hsa_ad=678431104790&hsa_ver=3&hsa_grp=154207406119&hsa_src=g&hsa_acc=2567925476&hsa_tgt=kwd-374487233417&gad_source=1&gclid=CjwKCAiA1-6sBhAoEiwArqlG-Pq2DAbIkhYbZhgsTeOGccrDjngQ4spE9xlx6jJSYCvdGxw0tLY9vQBoC-3Z0QAvD_BwE. Accessed 2024 Jan 8.

12. Crossley GH, Boyle A, Vitense H, Chang Y, Mead RH. The CONNECT (Clinical Evaluation of Remote Notification to Reduce Time to Clinical Decision) trial: the value of wireless remote monitoring with automatic clinician alerts. *J Am Coll Cardiol*. 2011;57:1181–1189.

13. Slotwiner D, Varma N, Akar JG, Annas G, Beardsall M, Fogel RI, et al. HRS expert consensus statement on remote interrogation and monitoring for cardiovascular implantable electronic devices. *Heart Rhythm*. 2015; 12:e69–e100.

14. Bayoumy K, Gaber M, Elshafeey A, Mhaimeed O, Dineen EH, Marvel FA, et al. Smart wearable devices in cardiovascular care: where we are and how to move forward. *Nat Rev Cardiol*. 2021;18:581–599. doi:10.1038/s41569-021-00522-7.

15. Rathbone AL, Prescott J. The use of mobile apps and SMS messaging as physical and mental health interventions: systematic review. *J Med Internet Res*. 2017 Aug 24;19(8):e295. doi:10.2196/jmir.7740.

16. Pearson AL, Mack E, Namanya J. Mobile phones and mental well-being: initial evidence suggesting the importance of staying connected to family in rural, remote communities in Uganda. *PLoS One*. 2017;12(1):e0169819. doi:10.1371/journal.pone.0169819.

17. Number of Mobile Phone Users Worldwide from 2015 to 2020 (in Billions). Statista. 2016. https://www.statista.com/statistics/274774/forecast-of-mobile-phone-users-worldwide/

18. Mobile Fact Sheet. Pew Research Center. 2024. http://www.pewinternet.org/fact-sheet/mobile/an.

19. Phaneuf A. The Number of Health and Fitness App Users Increased 27% from Last Year. Insider Intelligence. 2020. https://www.insiderintelligence.com/content/number-of-health-fitness-app-users-increased-27-last-year.

20. Brzan PP, Rotman E, Pajnkihar M, Klanjsek P. Mobile applications for control and self management of diabetes: a systematic review. *J Med Syst*. 2016 Sep;40(9):210. doi:10.1007/s10916-016-0564-8.

21. Policy for Device Software Functions and Mobile Medical Applications Guidance for Industry and Food and Drug Administration Staff. Silver Spring: U.S. Food & Drug Administration. 2022. https://www.fda.gov/regulatory-information/search-fda-guidance-documents/policy-device-software-functions-and-mobile-medical-applications.

22. Van Ameringen M, Turna J, Khalesi Z, Pullia K, Patterson B. There is an app for that! The current state of mobile applications (apps) for DSM-5 obsessive-compulsive disorder, posttraumatic stress disorder, anxiety and mood disorders. *Depress Anxiety*. 2017 Jun;34(6):526–539. doi:10.1002/da.22657.

23. Kampmeijer R, Pavlova M, Tambor M, Golinowska S, Groot W. The use of e-health and m-health tools in health promotion and primary prevention among older adults: a systematic literature review. *BMC Health Serv Res*. 2016 Sep 5;16(Suppl 5):290. doi:10.1186/s12913-016-1522-3.

24. Boulos MN, Wheeler S, Tavares C, Jones R. How smartphones are changing the face of mobile and participatory healthcare: an overview, with example from eCAALYX. *Biomed Eng*. 2011Apr 5;10:24. doi:10.1186/1475-925X-10-24.

25. Ahmed I, Ahmad NS, Ali S, Ali S, George A, Saleem Danish H et al. Medication adherence apps: review and content analysis. *JMIR Mhealth Uhealth*. 2018 Mar 16;6(3):e62. doi:10.2196/mhealth.6432.

26. Cano Martín JA, Martínez-Pérez B, de la Torre-Díez I, López-Coronado M. Economic impact assessment from the use of a mobile app for the self-management of heart diseases by patients with heart failure in a Spanish region. *J Med Syst*. 2014Sep;38(9):96. doi:10.1007/s10916-014-0096-z.

27. Chaudhry BM. Heart rate monitoring mobile applications. *Mhealth*. 2016 Apr 22;2:17. doi:10.21037/mhealth.2016.04.01. PMID: 28293594; PMCID: PMC5344133.

28. Ventola CL. Mobile devices and apps for mobile devices health care professionals: uses and benefits. *P T*. 2014 May;39(5):356–364. PMID: 24883008; PMCID: PMC4029126.

29. Ahn DT, Stahl R. Is there an app for that? The pros and cons of diabetes smartphone apps and how to integrate them into clinical practice. *Diabetes Spectr*. 2019 Aug;32(3):231–236. doi:10.2337/ds18-0101. PMID: 31462879; PMCID: PMC6695256.

30. Chandrashekar P. Do mental health mobile apps work: evidence and recommendations for designing high-efficacy mental health mobile apps. *Mhealth*. 2018Mar 23;4:6. doi:10.21037/mhealth.2018.03.02. PMID: 29682510; PMCID: PMC5897664.

31. Myfitnesspal. https://www.myfitnesspal.com/. Accessed 2024 Jan 7.

32. Headspace. https://www.headspace.com/newyear?utm_source=google& utm_medium=search&utm_campaign=HS_Headspace_Brand-Exact_ Search_US-NorAm_Google_NA&utm_content=&utm_term= headspace&gad_source=1&gclid=Cj0KCQiAtOmsBhCnARIsAGPa5yb6pv IlFCzaDKmeh4Kw7U6ZpOONdii2gX-s4DWkjyjir1Av1qlIVCUaAspgEALw_ wcB. Accessed 2024 Jan 7.

33. Teladoc. https://www.teladoc.com/start/?utm_medium=sem&utm_ source=google&utm_campaign=sem_google_th_enr_us_fm_web-mobile_ brand_bob_gen_ecpc_event3&utm_content=&utm_term=telado c_e_12009158636_115657028803_kwd-2843133695&pk_source=google& pk_medium=sem&pk_campaign=sem_google_th_enr_us_fm_web-mobile_ brand_bob_gen_ecpc_event3&gclid=Cj0KCQiAtOmsBhCnARIsAGPa5ya B46HHyHZGooV1yb0aq3euFAeOP9Ox1HAwFB- fBjXNsF2EpcoxxmEaAh-4EALw_wcB. Accessed 2024 Jan 7.

34. Torous J, Roberts LW. Needed innovation in digital health and smartphone applications for mental health: transparency and trust. *JAMA Psychiat*. 2017 May 1;74(5):437–438. doi:10.1001/jamapsychiatry.2017.0262. PMID: 28384700.

35. Free C, Phillips G, Watson L, Galli L, Felix L, Edwards P et al. The effectiveness of mobile-health technologies to improve health care service delivery processes: a systematic review and meta-analysis. *PLoS Med*. 2013;10(1):e1001363. doi:10.1371/journal.pmed.1001363. Epub 2013 Jan 15. PMID: 23458994; PMCID: PMC3566926.

36. Kuo DZ, McAllister JW, Rossignol L, Turchi RM, Stille CJ. Care coordination for children with medical complexity: whose care is it, anyway? *Pediatrics*. 2018 Mar;141(Suppl 3):S224–S232. doi:10.1542/peds.2017-1284G. PMID: 29496973.

37. Falconer E, Kho D, Docherty JP. Use of technology for care coordination initiatives for patients with mental health issues: a systematic literature review. *Neuropsychiatr Dis Treat*. 2018 Sep 13;14:2337–2349. doi:10.2147/NDT.S172810. PMID: 30254446; PMCID: PMC6143125.

38. Tabi K, Randhawa AS, Choi F, Mithani Z, Albers F, Schnieder M, et al. Mobile apps for medication management: review and analysis. *JMIR Mhealth Uhealth*. 2019 Sep 11;7(9):e13608. doi:10.2196/13608. PMID: 31512580; PMCID: PMC6786858.

39. Hightow-Weidman L, Muessig K, Knudtson K, Srivatsa M, Lawrence E, LeGrand S, et al. A gamified smartphone app to support engagement in care and medication adherence for HIV-positive young men who have sex with men (AllyQuest): development and pilot study. *JMIR Public Health Surveill*. 2018 Apr 30;4(2):e34. doi:10.2196/publichealth.8923.

40. Crosby LE, Ware RE, Goldstein A, Walton A, Joffe NE, Vogel C, et al. Development and evaluation of iManage: a self-management app co-designed by adolescents with sickle cell disease. *Pediatr Blood Cancer*. 2017 Jan;64(1):139–145. doi:10.1002/pbc.26177.

41. Anderson K, Burford O, Emmerton L. Mobile health apps to facilitate self-care: a qualitative study of user experiences. *PLoS One*. 2016;11(5):e0156164. doi:10.1371/journal.pone.0156164.

42. Morawski K, Ghazinouri R, Krumme A, Lauffenburger JC, Lu Z, Durfee E, et al. Association of a smartphone application with medication adherence and blood pressure control: the MedISAFE-BP randomized clinical trial. *JAMA Intern Med*. 2018 Jun 1;178(6):802–809. doi:10.1001/jamainternmed.2018.0447. Erratum in: *JAMA Intern Med*. 2018 Jun 1;178(6):876. PMID: 29710289; PMCID: PMC6145760.

43. Medisafe. https://www.medisafe.com/. Accessed 2024 Jan 6.

44. MyTherapy. https://www.mytherapyapp.com/. Accessed 2024 Jan 6.

45. Pérez-Jover V, Sala-González M, Guilabert M, Mira JJ. Mobile apps for increasing treatment adherence: systematic review. *J Med Internet Res*. 2019 Jun 18;21(6):e12505. doi:10.2196/12505. PMID: 31215517; PMCID: PMC6604503.

46. Al-Arkee S, Mason J, Lane DA, Fabritz L, Chua W, Haque MS, et al. Mobile apps to improve medication adherence in cardiovascular disease: systematic review and meta-analysis. *J Med Internet Res*. 2021 May 25;23(5):e24190. doi:10.2196/24190. PMID: 34032583; PMCID: PMC8188316.

47. Bodenheimer T, Lorig K, Holman H, Grumbach K. Patient self-management of chronic disease in primary care. *JAMA*. 2002;288:2469–2475. doi:10.1001/jama.288.19.2469

48. Grady PA, Gough LL. Self-management: a comprehensive approach to management of chronic conditions. *Am J Public Health*. 2014;104:e25–e31. doi:10.2105/AJPH.2014.302041

49. Quinn CC, Shardell MD, Terrin ML, Barr EA, Ballew SH, Gruber-Baldini AL. Cluster-randomized trial of a mobile phone personalized behavioral intervention for blood glucose control. *Diabetes Care*. 2011 Sep;34(9):1934–1942. doi:10.2337/dc11-0366. Epub 2011 Jul 25. Erratum in: *Diabetes Care*. 2013 Nov;36(11):3850. PMID: 21788632; PMCID: PMC3161305.

50. Zhai Y., Yu W. A mobile app for diabetes management: impact on self-efficacy among patients with type 2 diabetes at a community hospital. *Med Sci Monit*. 2020;26:e926719. doi: 10.12659/MSM.926719.

51. Whitehead L, Seaton P. The effectiveness of self-management mobile phone and tablet apps in long-term condition management: a systematic review. *J Med Internet Res*. 2016;18:e97. doi: 10.2196/jmir.4883.

52. Devan H, Farmery D, Peebles L, Grainger R. Evaluation of self-management support functions in apps for people with persistent pain: systematic review. *JMIR Mhealth Uhealth*. 2019;7:e13080. doi:10.2196/13080.

53. Hibbard, JH, Greene, J. What the evidence shows about patient activation: better health outcomes and care experiences; fewer data on costs. *Health Aff*. 2013;32:207–214. doi:10.1377/hlthaff.2012.1061.

54. WebMD. https://www.webmd.com/. Accessed 2024 Jan 6.

55. Symptomate. https://symptomate.com/. Accessed 2024 Jan 6.

56. Elwyn G, Coulter A, Laitner S, Walker E, Watson P, Thomson R. Implementing shared decision making in the NHS. *BMJ*. 2010;341:c5146. doi:10.1136/bmj.c5146

57. Ryan R, Deci E. Self-determination theory and the facilitation of intrinsic motivation, social development, and well-being. *Am Psychol*. 2000;55(1):68–78. doi:10.1037/0003-066X.55.1.68.

58. Entwistle VA, Carter SM, Cribb A, McCaffery K. Supporting patient autonomy: the importance of clinician-patient relationships. *J Gen Intern Med*. 2010;25(7):741–745. doi:10.1007/s11606-010-1292-2.

59. Elwyn G, Frosch D, Thomson R, Joseph-Williams N, Lloyd A, Kinnersley P, et al. Shared decision making: a model for clinical practice. *J Gen Intern Med*. 2012 Oct;27(10):1361–1367. doi:10.1007/s11606-012-2077-6. Epub 2012 May 23. PMID: 22618581; PMCID: PMC3445676.

60 Stacey D, Légaré F, Col NF, Lewis K, Barry MJ, Bennett CL, et al. Decision aids for people facing health treatment or screening decisions. *Cochrane Database Syst Rev.* 2014 Jan 28;1:CD001431. PMID: 24470076.

61. Da Silva D. *Evidence: Helping People Share Decisions. A Review of Evidence Considering Whether Shared Decision Making Is Worthwhile.* London: Health Foundation; 2012 June. http://www.health.org.uk/public/cms/75/76/313/3448/HelpingPeopleShareDecisionMaking.pdf?realName=rFVU5h.pd.

62. Wilson SR, Strub P, Buist AS, Knowles SB, Lavori PW, Lapidus J, et al. Shared treatment decision making improves adherence and outcomes in poorly controlled asthma. *Am J Respir Crit Care Med.* 2010 Mar 15;181(6):566–577. PMID: 20019345.

63. Zapata BC, Fernández-Alemán JL, Idri A, Toval A. Empirical studies on usability of mHealth apps: a systematic literature review. *J Med Syst.* 2015 Feb;39(2):1. doi:10.1007/s10916-014-0182-2. Epub 2015 Jan 20. PMID: 25600193.

Chapter 5

Genomics for Personalized Medicine

Introduction to Genomics and Personalized Medicine

This chapter explores the groundbreaking realms of genomics and personalized medicine, two fields at the forefront of modern healthcare innovation. Genomics, the extensive study of an organism's entire genetic code, delves deep into the complexities of genes, their interactions, and the influence of both environmental and lifestyle factors on these genetic blueprints. This comprehensive understanding paves the way for personalized medicine, a revolutionary approach that tailors healthcare to individual patients. By integrating genetic, environmental, and lifestyle data, personalized medicine aims to optimize treatment efficacy, minimize adverse drug reactions (ADRs), and open doors to preventive health strategies. This shift from a one-size-fits-all methodology to a more customized approach has profound implications for patient care. It enhances our understanding of disease processes and individual health risks and revolutionizes how treatments are prescribed and administered. As we navigate through this chapter, we will uncover how integrating genomics into clinical practice is not just transforming medical treatments but also redefining our approach to healthcare, making it more precise, predictive, and preventive. This chapter introduces these dynamic fields, highlighting their potential to align medical care more closely with each patient's unique genetic makeup.

Genomics: Scope and Basic Concepts

Genomics is the study of genomes, which includes all genetic material in an organism, encompassing DNA sequence, structure, function, evolution, and mapping. This field aims to understand an organism's complete set of genetic instructions and how these instructions influence its biology and health. The work of Lander et al.[1] in the Human Genome Project (HGP) exemplifies structural genomics, focusing on mapping and sequencing genetic information. Critical concepts in genomics include DNA sequencing, the process of determining the order of nucleotides within a DNA molecule.[2] Genetic variation, particularly single nucleotide polymorphisms (SNPs), is crucial for understanding genetic predisposition to diseases and drug responses.[3] Gene expression, the process by which instructions in DNA are converted into a functional product such as a protein, is essential for understanding the role of genes in health and disease.[4]

Genomics is a broad and interdisciplinary[5] field that includes structural genomics, functional genomics, pharmacogenomics, comparative genomics, and epigenomics.

Structural genomics deals with the organization and sequence of genetic information. Researchers in structural genomics examine the three-dimensional structures of proteins encoded by genes.[6,7] This field encompasses the mapping and sequencing of an organism's entire genome, both genetically and physically. The primary objective of structural genomics is to determine the structures of all unique protein folds experimentally.

Functional genomics investigates the functions and interactions of genes and proteins, understanding how DNA sequences result in biological functions.[8] This field focuses on understanding the roles and interactions of genes and proteins across the entire genome. It employs comprehensive, genome-wide methods, moving beyond the traditional approach of studying individual genes one at a time, as seen in classical molecular biology.

Pharmacogenomics, a part of functional genomics, exemplifies the application of genomics in medicine. This field combines pharmacology and genomics to develop effective, safe medications and doses tailored to a person's genetic makeup.[9] Indeed, the National Center for Biotechnology Information (NCBI) defines the term pharmacogenomics as "a science that examines the inherited variations in genes that dictate drug response and explores the ways these variations can be used to predict whether a patient will have a good response to a drug, a bad response to a drug, or no response at all."[10] Pharmacogenomics aims to tailor therapeutic strategies for individual patients, leveraging insights into human genome variability and its impact on drug efficacy to enhance treatment outcomes.[11]

Comparative genomics is a branch of biology where scientists employ diverse techniques to analyze and compare the entire genomic sequences of different species.[12] Through a detailed examination of traits that distinguish various organisms, researchers identify areas of both similarity and divergence. This science is sometimes used to shed light on evolutionary processes.[13]

Epigenomics

The term "epigenome" is derived from the Greek word "epi," which translates to "above" in relation to the genome. It comprises chemical compounds that bind to the genome and play a crucial role in regulating its functions. These compounds determine when, where, and how the genetic instructions are executed. Each cell type possesses a distinct set of these epigenetic marks, which are separate from the DNA sequence itself. These marks can be transmitted from one cell generation to the next and can even be passed down through generations.

Epigenomics is the study of these epigenetic modifications, focusing on changes in gene expression that occur without altering the underlying DNA sequence.[14] Previously, the scientific consensus was that human diseases primarily stemmed from alterations in DNA sequences, infections by agents such as bacteria and viruses, or exposure to environmental factors. However, recent research has shown that modifications in the epigenome can also be a cause or a consequence of various diseases. Fundamental mechanisms driving these modifications include DNA methylation, chromatin modifications, loss of imprinting, and the actions of noncoding RNA. These mechanisms differ from mutations, which involve direct changes to the DNA sequence.

This aspect of epigenetics explains why identical twins, who inherit the same genes from their parents, can exhibit differences in physical traits, behaviors, and disease risks. Despite sharing the same genetic code, the variations in their epigenomes can lead to different gene expression patterns, resulting in these observable differences.[15]

Milestones in Genomics

The field of genomics has witnessed several pivotal milestones. In 1953, Watson and Crick's[16] discovery of the DNA double helix laid the foundational framework for understanding genetic information. This was followed by the Human Genome Project, completed in 2003, which mapped the entire human genome, providing a comprehensive reference for human genetic variation.[17]

Another significant advancement was the development of next-generation sequencing (NGS) technologies.[18] NGS, or high-throughput sequencing, refers to advanced sequencing technologies that have revolutionized genomic research. Traditionally, genetic testing was available for few genes because sequencing depended on the Sanger-based (dideoxy) DNA method,[19] the gold standard for detecting mutations at the base pair level. The Sanger method sequenced one strand of DNA at a time, which was slow and expensive. Unlike first-generation Sanger sequencing, NGS allows for the simultaneous sequencing of millions of DNA fragments, dramatically increasing the speed and reducing the cost of sequencing.

These technologies, emerging prominently in the early 21st century, have drastically reduced the cost and time required for genomic sequencing, making it more accessible for research and clinical applications.[20]

Integration of Genomics into Medical Practice

Integrating genomics into medical practice has been transformative, particularly in personalized medicine and pharmacogenomics. Genomic approaches have significantly impacted medical practice in various areas.[21] In prevention, they are used for noninvasive prenatal testing, expanded carrier screening for genetic disorders, and assessing the risk of common diseases. In pharmacogenomics, genetic information predicts an individual's response to drugs, optimizing drug efficacy and minimizing adverse effects. A well-known example is the use of the thiopurine methyltransferase (TPMT) gene test before prescribing azathioprine. This test helps to identify patients at risk of severe side effects due to TPMT deficiency.

Diagnostic advancements include cytogenomics and the use of whole-exome or -genome sequencing. In therapeutics, pharmacogenetic testing, tumor genome sequencing for cancer treatment and the development of targeted therapies are notable applications. For example, in oncology, genomic testing is routinely used to identify specific mutations in cancer cells. This information guides the selection of targeted therapies, improving treatment efficacy and reducing side effects. A notable instance is the use of trastuzumab in HER2-positive breast cancer patients, a treatment decision based on genomic testing.[22]

While advances in human genomics are ushering in a new era of predictive, preventative, and personalized approaches to medicine, its integration into medical practice is not without challenges.[23,24] The large size and complexity of genetic test results, the lack of standardized clinical and genetic data, and the limitations of EHR systems in storing and analyzing genetic data are obstacles. Additionally, there are concerns about interpreting regulations regarding the return of genetic test results and privacy issues specific to genetic data.[25] Public access to their genomic data gives many healthcare providers pause. Many healthcare professionals have reservations about direct-to-consumer genomic profiling due to concerns about the clinical validity of these tests. Additionally, there is worry that patients might misinterpret the results without proper medical guidance, which could lead to psychological distress or impact their well-being.[26–28]

There are also ethical considerations[29] in dealing with genomic data. For example, when genomic data are publicly accessible, there is a risk of discrimination in getting jobs or health insurance if genomic data suggest a risk of cancer, chronic disease, or mental illness. With all its new clinical possibilities, healthcare professionals need to stay abreast of rapidly evolving genomic knowledge.[30]

Healthcare professionals are tasked with effectively conveying genomic data to patients,[31] including several vital aspects.[32] First, they must address the uncertainties inherent in genomic data, particularly when no therapeutic course of action exists. This involves evaluating and communicating the implications of both positive and negative test results, even when these results do not definitively predict the development of a disease from a gene variant. Additionally, professionals must adeptly translate broad population screening statistics into meaningful, individualized information for each patient. Finally, they must be prepared to counteract potential biases that may arise from misinterpretations in the popular media or overstatements by the scientific community.

The potential of genomics to revolutionize healthcare is immense, promising more precise, predictive, and personalized medical care. While routine genome sequencing for all individuals is possible, it faces technical, ethical, and medical system challenges. Integrating genomics into medical practice will be a gradual but ongoing process.

The Transformative Potential of Genomics

Overview of Advancements

Genomics has significantly advanced in recent years, fundamentally altering our understanding of health and disease. Key advancements include high-throughput sequencing technologies, which have made genome sequencing faster and more affordable.[18] This has improved diagnostic capabilities, particularly in identifying rare genetic disorders and characterizing cancers at the molecular level.[33] Sometimes, this testing reveals unexpected findings. The American College of Medical Genetics and Genomics (ACMG) has acknowledged the potential for incidental or secondary findings in clinical exome and genome sequencing, which are unrelated to the primary reason for testing but may have medical value. They emphasize the importance of informing patients about the possibility of such findings during pretest discussions, testing, and result reporting. The ACMG formed a working group to develop guidelines for managing these incidental findings. After a year-long consensus process, including public forums and expert reviews, this group recommended that laboratories performing clinical sequencing should actively look for and report specific mutations in specified genes. The ACMG acknowledges the need for more comprehensive data on the penetrance and clinical utility of these findings and advocates for regular updates to these recommendations as more data become available.

Another major advancement is in pharmacogenomics, where genetic information guides drug development and prescription, thus reducing adverse drug reactions and increasing efficacy.[9] Pharmacogenomics represents a significant advancement in personalized medicine, leveraging genetic information to guide drug development and prescription. This approach aims to optimize drug efficacy and minimize adverse drug reactions, a major concern in clinical practice. Indeed, the field of pharmacogenetics developed only after the variation in drug responses was attributed to large single-gene effects.[34,35]

Pharmacogenomics integrates the study of how genes affect a person's drug response. This is based on the understanding that genetic variations can affect individual responses to medications, influencing how well a drug works or how likely it is to cause side effects. For example, variations in the CYP450 family of enzymes, which are responsible for metabolizing many drugs, can significantly alter a patient's response to a wide range of medications, including antidepressants and statins.[36]

Pharmacogenomics aids in identifying novel drug targets and designing drugs with increased specificity. This can lead to the development of more effective therapies with fewer side effects than traditional drugs. For instance, the development of targeted cancer therapies, such as trastuzumab for HER2-positive breast cancer, is a direct result of pharmacogenomic research.[22]

In clinical practice, pharmacogenomic testing can inform prescribing decisions. For example, testing for HLA-B*5701 can prevent hypersensitivity reactions in patients treated with abacavir, an antiretroviral drug.[37] Additionally, warfarin dosing can be refined based on VKORC1 and CYP2C9 genotypes to reduce the risk of bleeding or thrombosis.[38]

However, challenges remain in integrating pharmacogenomics into routine clinical practice. These include the need for more comprehensive studies to establish the clinical utility of pharmacogenomic tests, developing guidelines for interpreting test results and integrating these tests into clinical workflows.[39]

Future Prospects in Healthcare

The future of genomics in healthcare is promising, with potential impacts across various domains. One area is predictive medicine, where genomic information could be used to predict a patient's disease risk and implement early interventions.[40] For example, genetic testing for BRCA1/2 mutations, which are linked to an increased risk of breast and ovarian cancers, allows for personalized monitoring and preventive measures, such as increased surveillance or prophylactic surgeries.[41]

Another area of impact is pharmacogenomics, which involves tailoring drug therapies based on an individual's genetic makeup to maximize efficacy and minimize adverse reactions. For instance, genotyping for the TPMT enzyme can guide the dosing of thiopurines in treating leukemia, reducing the risk of severe side effects.[42]

Additionally, genomics can play a role in diagnosing rare genetic disorders. Techniques such as whole-exome sequencing, which sequences the genome's protein-coding regions, have been instrumental in identifying rare genetic mutations in patients with undiagnosed diseases.[43] The protein-coding regions account for about 1–2% of the human genome but contain about 85% of known disease-related variants.[44,45] This technique particularly effectively identifies rare genetic mutations often missed by traditional diagnostic methods.

Another prospect is the integration of genomics with emerging technologies such as AI and machine learning (ML), which could enhance the interpretation of complex genetic data and improve diagnostic and personalized treatment accuracy.[46]

AI and ML algorithms can process and analyze vast amounts of genomic data at a speed and accuracy unattainable by human clinicians. The complexity and sheer volume of data produced by contemporary genomic methods, such as whole genome sequencing, necessitate advanced analysis techniques. AI is pivotal in this context. AI, particularly through its subsets ML and deep learning (DL), is adept at processing and interpreting the vast amounts of genetic data generated. These AI algorithms excel at detecting patterns, making predictions, and categorizing genetic variations, leveraging their ability to learn from extensive datasets. For example, AI can uncover patterns and associations within genetic data that might indicate the presence of specific diseases, a task that is challenging to perform manually.

AI-driven tools are revolutionizing the diagnosis of rare genetic diseases by accurately identifying the specific genetic mutations responsible for a patient's condition, even when there are thousands of possible mutations. Currently, the Online Mendelian Inheritance in Man (OMIM) database lists about 10,000 monogenic disorders, diseases caused by mutations in a single gene, at the level of their symptoms or phenotypes. However, the gene responsible for less than half of these diseases has been identified. AI in this field can significantly accelerate the diagnosis of these rare diseases. For example, AI has been instrumental in determining the genetic basis of disorders such as spinocerebellar ataxia, a rare, genetically heterogeneous disease that causes progressive gait difficulties due to degeneration of the cerebellum, corticospinal tracts, brainstem, and spinal cord. AI has been able to determine the causes by analyzing genetic variations from a large dataset of patients.[47-49] This rapid and precise identification can significantly reduce the time and complexity involved in reaching a diagnosis for patients with rare genetic conditions.

In rare genetic diseases, AI-driven tools can assist in pinpointing the exact genetic mutations responsible for a patient's condition, often from among thousands of potential candidates. Today, around 10,000 monogenic disorders are listed in the OMIM database at the phenotypic level. However, the genes responsible for these diseases have been identified in less than half of these cases. This rapid identification can significantly shorten the diagnostic odyssey for patients with rare diseases.

Cancer Genomics

The efficacy of cancer therapies is profoundly influenced by a range of factors, including the tumor's genetic profile, its microenvironment, the likelihood of developing resistance to drugs, and the principles of pharmacogenomics.[50] The genetic diversity of tumors among different patients, which leads to variations in protein expression, highlights the critical need for personalized and precision approaches in cancer treatment.[51]

Cancer genomics is a specialized field within genomics focusing on the study of genes associated with cancer.[52] It involves identifying oncogenes and tumor-suppressor genes that are crucial for clinical diagnostics. In cancer genomics, AI and ML are increasingly vital. These technologies are essential in deepening our understanding of tumors' genetic and biological aspects, enabling the development of more personalized treatment plans. By analyzing tumor genetic data, AI and ML can identify specific mutations and predict the most effective treatment options for individual patients. This approach is at the heart of precision oncology, which focuses on customizing cancer treatment based on the unique genetic makeup of each patient's tumor, moving away from generic treatment protocols.[53]

AI algorithms, for example, can detect genetic variations within tumor DNA that may be critical in cancer progression.[53,54] This information is invaluable for oncologists in choosing targeted therapies that are more likely to be successful based on the patient's unique genetic profile. AI and ML are also instrumental in forecasting patient responses to different cancer treatments. A case in point is the use of AI in lung cancer, where these technologies aid in understanding the genomic pathways by optimizing algorithms.[55,56] AI classifiers, an algorithm used in AI and ML, can predict cancer subtypes, tumor growth, and the likelihood of metastasis.[57] As NGS and other techniques advance, enabling more detailed insights into gene expression patterns, clinicians can increasingly use genomic data to make personalized treatment decisions.[58]

Moreover, AI's ability to detect a high mutational burden in tumor genomes has been associated with improved responses to checkpoint inhibitors in treating non-small cell lung cancer.[59]

Additionally, AI and ML's contributions to pharmacogenomics are significant. They aid in predicting individual responses to drugs based on genetic factors. This progress is leading to more effective and safer drug prescriptions, reducing the trial-and-error approach often associated with determining the right medication for a patient.

Another area where these technologies are making an impact is the emerging field of precision public health, which leverages genomic data to tailor public health interventions to specific groups. However, integrating AI and ML in healthcare is challenging, including ethical considerations, data privacy issues, and the need for healthcare systems to adapt to these rapidly advancing technologies.

Genomic Testing and Therapy Selection

Understanding Genomic Tests

Genomic testing, a cornerstone of personalized medicine, involves analyzing an individual's DNA to gain insights into their genetic makeup. This testing plays a pivotal role in guiding therapy selection, offering a more tailored approach to treatment.

Types of Genomic Tests

There are several types of genomic tests, each serving different purposes in the context of healthcare:

Diagnostic Testing

Diagnostic testing in genetics is a critical tool used to identify or confirm the presence of a specific genetic or chromosomal condition. This type of testing is often employed when a genetic disorder is suspected based on physical symptoms, family history, or the results of other medical tests.

A prominent example of diagnostic testing is the analysis of BRCA1 and BRCA2 genes for assessing breast cancer risk.[60] Mutations in these genes are known to significantly increase the risk of developing breast and ovarian cancers. Women with harmful mutations in BRCA1 or BRCA2 have a risk of breast cancer that is about 5 times the average risk and a risk of ovarian cancer that is about 10–30 times normal. Identifying a BRCA mutation can be crucial for making informed decisions about preventive measures, such as enhanced screening, prophylactic surgery, or chemoprevention.

Diagnostic genetic testing isn't limited to cancer risk assessment. It encompasses a wide range of genetic disorders, including cystic fibrosis, sickle cell anemia, Huntington's disease, and many others. The testing process typically involves collecting a sample of blood, skin, amniotic fluid (in prenatal testing), or other tissue and analyzing the DNA contained in the cells.

The results from diagnostic genetic testing can have significant implications for an individual's healthcare management. For instance, identifying a specific genetic mutation can guide healthcare providers in choosing the most effective treatment and management strategies. It can also provide valuable information for family planning and risk assessment for family members.

It's important to note that while diagnostic testing can provide crucial information about genetic risks, it also raises ethical and psychological considerations, such as the impact of knowing one's genetic predisposition to a severe illness. Therefore, genetic counseling is often recommended alongside diagnostic testing to help individuals understand the test results' implications and support them in making informed decisions.

Predictive and Presymptomatic Testing

Predictive and presymptomatic genetic testing are genetic analyses used to assess the risk of developing a specific genetic disorder before any symptoms are evident. This form of testing is particularly relevant for individuals with a known family history of a genetic condition but who currently show no symptoms of the disorder.

One classic example of this testing is for Huntington's disease, a progressive brain disorder caused by a single defective gene on chromosome 4. This defect is a specific kind of mutation called a trinucleotide repeat.[61] Typically, this DNA segment varies from person to person, but individuals with Huntington's disease have a higher number of repeats, leading to the disease's development. Predictive testing for Huntington's disease can determine whether an individual has inherited this mutation and consequently will develop the condition later in life.

The implications of predictive and presymptomatic testing are profound. For at-risk individuals, these tests can clarify their future health and enable them to make informed decisions about their life and medical care. For instance, someone who tests positive for the Huntington's disease gene might choose to pursue specific life goals earlier or differently than they might have otherwise. They might also make specific healthcare or financial plans to accommodate their future needs.

However, these tests also raise significant psychological and ethical issues. Learning that one is likely to develop a serious, potentially debili-tating condition later in life can be distressing and may have mental health implications. Moreover, there are considerations regarding insurance dis-crimination and the privacy of genetic information. Therefore, genetic counseling is strongly recommended alongside predictive and presympto-matic testing. Genetic counselors can provide information, support, and guidance to individuals and families undergoing these tests, helping them to understand the results and their implications.

Carrier Testing

Carrier testing is a type of genetic testing used to determine whether an individual carries a gene mutation associated with certain inherited disorders.[62] This testing is essential for disorders that follow an autosomal recessive inheritance pattern, where a person must inherit two copies of the mutated gene (one from each parent) to manifest the disease. Individuals who carry only one copy of the mutated gene typically do not show symptoms of the disorder but have a chance of passing the gene to their offspring.

One of the most well-known applications of carrier testing is screen-ing for cystic fibrosis (CF). CF is a life-threatening disorder caused by mutations in the cystic fibrosis transmembrane conductance regulator (CFTR) gene. It causes severe damage to the lungs, digestive system, and other organs. Carrier testing for CF involves analyzing an individual's DNA to check for mutations in the CFTR gene. This is particularly rele-vant for people with a family history of CF or partners of CF carriers.

If both parents are carriers of a CF mutation, there is a 25% chance with each pregnancy that the child will have CF, a 50% chance that the child will be a carrier, and a 25% chance that the child will neither have CF nor be a carrier.

Carrier testing is also available for other genetic conditions, such as sickle cell anemia, Tay–Sachs disease, and thalassemia. It is often recom-mended for individuals or couples who are planning to start a family and want to be informed about the risk of having a child with a genetic disorder.

The results of carrier testing can provide valuable information for making informed decisions about family planning. They can also guide discussions with healthcare providers about managing potential risks in future pregnancies.

Pharmacogenomic Testing

An unsettling fact for prescribers is that 20–75% of patients may fail to respond to many commonly used drugs.[63] This variation in response has spurred the development of pharmacogenomic testing. Pharmacogenomic testing represents a critical intersection between genetics and pharmacology, focusing on how an individual's genetic makeup influences their medication response.[64] This form of testing is gaining prominence as a tool for personalized medicine, aiming to optimize drug efficacy and minimize adverse reactions.

The variability in drug responses among different individuals is a significant challenge in medical treatment. While a particular medication may be effective and safe for one person, it can cause severe adverse reactions or be utterly ineffective in yet another. This variability can be primarily attributed to genetic differences, estimated to account for approximately 20–95% of the variation in drug responses.[65] These genetic differences can affect drug metabolism, efficacy, and the likelihood of adverse effects.

Pharmacogenomic testing, such as warfarin sensitivity testing, exemplifies the practical application of this concept. Warfarin, a commonly prescribed anticoagulant, requires careful dosing to ensure effectiveness while avoiding potentially dangerous bleeding complications. Genetic variations in enzymes, such as CYP2C9 and VKORC1, significantly influence how individuals metabolize warfarin.[39] By testing for these genetic variants, physicians can tailor warfarin doses more precisely, enhancing treatment safety and effectiveness.

Beyond warfarin, pharmacogenomics has applications across a wide range of drugs, including chemotherapy agents, antidepressants, and statins. For example, specific genetic variants can predict how a patient will respond to specific chemotherapy drugs, allowing oncologists to choose a treatment plan with a higher likelihood of success and fewer side effects.

Implementing pharmacogenomic testing in clinical practice can significantly improve drug therapy management. It enables healthcare providers to select the most appropriate medications and dosages for individual patients based on their genetic profiles, thus reducing the trial-and-error approach often associated with medication prescribing.

However, integrating pharmacogenomics into routine clinical practice also presents challenges, including the need for more extensive genetic education among healthcare providers, the development of guidelines for interpreting test results, and considerations regarding the cost and accessibility of testing.

Genomic Testing: Mechanisms and Technologies Involved

The mechanisms and technologies underpinning genomic testing have evolved significantly. They include NGS, polymerase chain reaction (PCR), and microarray technology.

Next-Generation Sequencing (NGS)

NGS has revolutionized genomic testing by enabling rapid, large-scale DNA sequencing, including whole-genome sequencing.[66] Following enhancements in accuracy, robustness, and usability, this method has become a widely adopted alternative to traditional Sanger sequencing.[67,68] Sanger sequencing could only process short DNA sequences at a time. At the same time, NGS allows for the simultaneous sequencing of millions of DNA fragments, significantly speeding up the genome sequencing process and reducing its cost.

NGS's impact is profound in both clinical and research settings.[69] The use of NGS in clinical laboratories has become increasingly common. It is now used to diagnose various conditions, including infectious diseases,[70] immune disorders,[71] and hereditary human disorders.[72] NGS is also employed in noninvasive prenatal diagnosis,[73] and more recently, has been instrumental in making therapeutic decisions for somatic cancers.[74]

In genetic research, NGS has proven to be a powerful tool for identifying new genes or variants linked to inherited diseases. This is particularly true for genetically heterogeneous disorders, where the genetic underpinnings were previously unclear, and a gene-by-gene Sanger sequencing approach would have needed to be more cost-effective and efficient.[75] NGS has been applied to whole-genome, -exome, or targeted sequencing, significantly enhancing our understanding of the genetic foundations of various diseases, including bronchopulmonary dysplasia,[76] hereditary retinal disorders,[77] and inherited cancers.[78]

However, NGS also brings challenges in data management and interpretation, requiring sophisticated computational resources and expertise in genetics and bioinformatics.[79] As NGS technology evolves, it is set to enhance medical diagnostics and personalized medicine further.

Polymerase Chain Reaction (PCR)

PCR is a pivotal technique in molecular biology and genomics that amplifies small DNA samples into quantities large enough for detailed analysis.[80] This method, developed in the 1980s, has become a fundamental tool in various biological research and medical diagnostics areas.[81]

The essence of PCR is its ability to take a minuscule amount of DNA and exponentially amplify it to millions or billions of copies. This amplification is achieved through a series of temperature changes in a process known as thermal cycling. The cycle typically involves denaturation (where the double-stranded DNA is separated into two single strands), annealing (where short DNA sequences known as primers bind to the single-stranded DNA), and extension (where a DNA polymerase enzyme synthesizes new strands of DNA complementary to the original strand).

PCR's versatility makes it invaluable in numerous genomic testing applications. In infectious diseases, PCR detects the presence of pathogen DNA or RNA in a patient's sample, which is crucial for diagnosing diseases such as HIV, tuberculosis, and COVID-19. In genetics, PCR is employed to identify specific genetic mutations, enabling the diagnosis of genetic disorders,[82] the detection of genetic markers in cancer, and even paternity testing.

The technique's sensitivity and specificity make it particularly useful when only trace amounts of DNA are available. This has led to its widespread use in forensic science for analyzing crime scene samples, in environmental biology for detecting low levels of pathogens in water or soil, and in paleobiology for studying ancient DNA samples.

PCR has also been instrumental in developing more advanced genomic technologies, including DNA sequencing and genotyping. Its ability to produce large quantities of a specific DNA segment makes it an essential step in many NGS protocols.[83]

Microarray Technology

Microarray technology is a genomics technique widely used for analyzing gene expression and single nucleotide polymorphism (SNP) genotyping.[84] Developed in the mid-1990s, microarrays allow for the simultaneous analysis of thousands of genes, providing a comprehensive snapshot of gene activity and genetic variations within an organism.

At its core, a microarray is a small, solid support — usually a glass slide or silicon chip — onto which DNA sequences are fixed in an orderly manner. Each spot on a microarray represents a different gene or a sequence of interest. In gene expression studies, microarrays are used to simultaneously measure the expression levels of large numbers of genes. This is achieved by comparing the amount of mRNA (which reflects gene activity) bound to each spot on the array. This method has been instrumental in understanding how gene expression changes under different conditions, such as in response to a drug treatment or in various stages of a disease.

To better understand SNP genotyping and microarrays, it's helpful first to review what SNPs are. A single nucleotide polymorphism, commonly abbreviated as SNP (pronounced "snip"), is a variation in a single nucleotide that occurs at a specific position in the genome. Nucleotides are the basic building blocks of DNA, consisting of adenine (A), thymine (T), cytosine (C), and guanine (G). In an SNP, one of these nucleotides is replaced by another at a particular DNA spot. For example, a DNA sequence might change from AAGGCTAA to ATGGCTAA, where the third nucleotide has changed from 'A' to 'T.' Most SNPs do not affect health or development, but some can play a significant role in influencing a person's disease risk, response to drugs, and other traits. Because of their abundance and distribution throughout the genome, SNPs are valuable in genetic research for locating genes associated with diseases, responses to drugs, and other health traits.

In SNP genotyping, microarrays identify variations at single nucleotide positions in the genome. Microarray technology simultaneously enables the analysis of thousands of SNPs, facilitating large-scale genetic association studies, population genetics research, and personalized medicine approaches.

Microarrays' ability to provide a vast amount of genetic information in a single experiment has made them invaluable in various fields of biological and medical research. They are used in cancer research to identify gene expression profiles associated with different types of tumors, in developmental biology to study gene expression patterns during organism development, and in pharmacogenomics to understand how genetic differences affect individual responses to drugs.

Microarray technology has evolved over the years, with advancements in data quality, array density, and analysis techniques. Despite the rise of NGS, microarrays remain a cost-effective and efficient tool for many genomic applications.

Genomics in Therapy Choices

Role in Drug Selection and Dosage

The integration of genomics into therapeutic decision-making has significantly enhanced the precision of drug selection and dosage. Pharmacogenomics, a branch of genomics, plays a crucial role in this process by examining how genetic variations affect individual responses to medications.[85,86] This approach enables healthcare providers to select drugs and dosages that are most likely to be effective and safe for each patient based on their genetic makeup.

For instance, certain genetic variations can influence how a patient metabolizes a drug. A well-known example is the variation in the CYP2C19 gene affecting the metabolism of clopidogrel, a commonly prescribed antiplatelet medication.[87] Patients with certain variants of this gene may require alternative medications or adjusted dosages to achieve the desired therapeutic effect. Similarly, variations in the VKORC1 and CYP2C9 genes influence warfarin sensitivity and dosage requirements, helping to mitigate the risk of bleeding or thrombosis.[88]

Impact on Treatment Efficacy

Genomic information can significantly impact the efficacy of treatments. By understanding the genetic factors that influence disease progression and drug response, clinicians can tailor treatments to the individual, thereby improving outcomes. In oncology, for example, genomic analysis of tumor DNA can identify specific mutations driving cancer growth. Targeted therapies, which are drugs developed to specifically counteract these mutations, can then be employed, often with greater success than conventional chemotherapy.

In chronic diseases such as diabetes and hypertension, genomics can help in predicting which patients are likely to benefit from certain medications, thus avoiding the trial-and-error approach often associated with these conditions.[89] This not only improves patient outcomes but also reduces the time and cost associated with finding the right medication.

Some studies have shown that even direct-to-consumer genomic profiling has been beneficial in identifying and preventing disease.[90]

The application of genomics in therapy choices marks a shift toward more personalized and effective healthcare.[91] By aligning drug selection and dosage with individual genetic profiles, genomics paves the way for treatments that are not only more effective but also carry fewer risks of adverse effects. This personalized approach is a cornerstone of modern precision medicine, offering hope for better patient outcomes across a wide range of diseases.

Avoiding Adverse Reactions through Genomics

Predictive Role of Genomic Testing

Genomic testing plays a critical role in predicting and preventing adverse drug reactions, enhancing the safety of medical treatments.[92] By understanding an individual's genetic makeup, healthcare providers can anticipate how they might react to certain medications, thus avoiding potential harmful effects.

Mechanisms of Adverse Drug Reactions

Adverse drug reactions are unintended, harmful events attributed to the use of medicines. They have become a frequent cause of morbidity and mortality[93] and an increasing challenge in modern healthcare, particularly given the increasing complexity of therapeutics, an aging population, and rising multimorbidity.[94] They can occur due to various mechanisms, often influenced by genetic factors. These mechanisms include altered drug metabolism, hypersensitivity reactions, and genetically predisposed toxicities. For example, some individuals have genetic variations that affect the function of liver enzymes responsible for drug metabolism. These variations can lead to either an accumulation of the drug to toxic levels or insufficient drug levels to be effective. Another example is the hypersensitivity to abacavir, a drug used in HIV treatment, which is strongly associated with the HLA-B*57:01 allele. Patients with this genetic variant are at a significantly increased risk of developing a severe hypersensitivity reaction to the drug.[95]

Genomic Predictors of Drug Response

Genomic predictors of drug response, often identified through pharmacogenomic testing, are genetic variations that influence an individual's response to a drug. These predictors can indicate whether a patient is likely to experience an adverse reaction or whether they will respond well to the treatment. For instance, variations in the TPMT gene can affect the response to thiopurine drugs, used in certain types of cancer and autoimmune diseases. Patients with certain TPMT gene mutations are at increased risk of toxicity from thiopurines due to reduced enzyme activity leading to drug accumulation.

By incorporating genomic testing into clinical practice, healthcare providers can identify patients at risk of adverse drug reactions and adjust medication choices and dosages accordingly.[96] This approach not only improves patient safety but also contributes to more effective and personalized treatment strategies. As genomic testing becomes more accessible and integrated into healthcare systems, it holds the promise of significantly reducing the incidence and severity of adverse drug reactions.

Tailoring Treatments for Improved Outcomes

Personalized Treatment Approaches

Personalized treatment approaches in medicine are grounded in the concept of tailoring healthcare to individual patients based on their unique genetic makeup, lifestyle, and environmental factors. This methodology represents a shift from the traditional one-size-fits-all approach to a more targeted strategy. It involves analyzing a patient's genetic profile to predict their response to various treatments and to identify any potential risk of adverse reactions.

The methodology of personalized treatment typically involves collecting and analyzing genetic data through methods such as genomic sequencing or SNP genotyping. This information is then integrated with clinical data, including the patient's medical history, current health status, and lifestyle factors. The combination of this data allows healthcare providers to develop a treatment plan that is more likely to be effective and less likely to cause side effects.

Genomic Tailoring in Practice

In practice, genomic tailoring is being applied in various medical fields with notable success. In oncology, for example, genomic analysis of tumors helps in identifying specific mutations that can be targeted by certain drugs, leading to the development of targeted therapies. A well-known example is the use of trastuzumab in breast cancer patients who overexpress the HER2 gene.

In pharmacogenomics, genetic testing is used to determine the right medication and dosage for patients. For instance, patients with certain genetic variants might metabolize drugs faster or slower than average, affecting the drug's efficacy and safety. By adjusting the drug type or dosage based on these genetic insights, clinicians can significantly improve treatment outcomes.

Another area where genomic tailoring is making an impact is in rare genetic disorders. By understanding the specific genetic mutations involved, treatments can be developed to target these mutations more precisely. This approach not only improves the efficacy of treatments but also reduces the time and resources spent on ineffective therapies.

The implementation of genomic tailoring in clinical practice is not without its challenges, including the need for advanced technology, skilled interpretation of genetic data, and considerations of cost and accessibility. However, the potential benefits it offers in terms of improved patient outcomes and more efficient healthcare delivery are substantial.

For instance, in cardiovascular medicine, genomic tailoring is used to identify patients at risk of adverse reactions to statins, a common cholesterol-lowering medication. By identifying genetic markers associated with these reactions, physicians can prescribe alternative treatments or adjust dosages accordingly.

In the field of mental health, genomic tailoring is beginning to inform the treatment of conditions such as depression and anxiety. Certain genetic markers can indicate how a patient might respond to antidepressants, allowing for more personalized treatment plans that are more likely to be effective and have fewer side effects.

Overall, the practice of genomic tailoring represents a significant advancement in the field of medicine. It embodies the principles of precision medicine, where treatments are based not just on the disease but also on the genetic and environmental factors unique to each individual. As research in this area continues to grow and technologies advance, the scope of genomic tailoring is expected to expand, further revolutionizing the approach to healthcare and treatment.

Outcome Analysis

Standard vs Personalized Treatment

The comparison between standard and personalized treatment approaches is pivotal in understanding the impact of genomics in clinical practice.

Standard treatments typically follow a generalized approach based on the average response of a large patient population. In contrast, personalized treatments, informed by genomic insights, are tailored to the individual characteristics of each patient.

A study highlighting this difference can be seen in cancer treatment. Traditional chemotherapy, a standard approach, often employs a one-size-fits-all regimen. However, personalized treatments, such as the use of trastuzumab for HER2-positive breast cancer patients, are based on the patient's specific genetic profile. Studies have shown that patients receiving trastuzumab, a targeted therapy, have significantly improved survival rates compared to those receiving standard chemotherapy alone.[97]

Long-term Benefits and Challenges

The long-term benefits of personalized treatment are substantial. They include improved efficacy of treatments, reduced incidence of adverse drug reactions, and potentially lower healthcare costs due to more effective therapies and fewer trial-and-error approaches. For instance, in the treatment of CF, the use of the drug ivacaftor in patients with specific CFTR mutations has led to notable improvements in lung function and quality of life.[98]

Current Barriers and Disparities to Equitable Access to Validated Pharmacogenomic Testing

Socioeconomic Factors

Socioeconomic factors play a significant role in creating disparities in access to pharmacogenomic testing. The cost of such testing can be prohibitive for individuals without adequate health insurance or those in lower socioeconomic groups. This financial barrier limits the availability of personalized medicine to a privileged few, exacerbating health inequalities. Additionally, there is often a lack of awareness or understanding of pharmacogenomics among populations with limited access to healthcare education, further widening the gap.

Healthcare System Limitations

The healthcare system itself presents limitations that can impede the widespread adoption of pharmacogenomic testing. These include a lack of standardized guidelines for when and how to use these tests, insufficient integration of pharmacogenomic data into electronic health records, and a shortage of healthcare professionals trained in interpreting and applying genomic information. Furthermore, the uneven distribution of advanced healthcare facilities capable of conducting such tests often leads to geographical disparities, where patients in rural or underserved areas have less access to these cutting-edge services.

Addressing these barriers requires a multifaceted approach, including policy changes to improve insurance coverage for pharmacogenomic testing, educational initiatives to raise awareness about its benefits, and investment in healthcare infrastructure and training. By tackling these issues, the healthcare system can move toward providing more equitable access to pharmacogenomic testing, ensuring that the benefits of personalized medicine are available to all segments of the population.

Ethical, Legal, and Social Implications of Genomic Medicine

Ethical Challenges

The integration of genomics into clinical medicine brings with it a host of ethical challenges, particularly concerning privacy, consent, and the potential for genetic discrimination. These issues require careful consideration to ensure ethical practices in the use of genomic information.

Privacy concerns in genomics primarily revolve around how genetic data are stored, shared, and used. The sensitive nature of genetic information, which can reveal predispositions to certain diseases or conditions, necessitates stringent privacy protections. For instance, the case of Henrietta Lacks, whose cancer cells were used to create an immortal cell line without her consent, highlights the importance of informed consent in genetic research.[99] The Lacks' family was distressed by the use of Henrietta's cells for scientific research for several reasons, primarily centered around the lack of consent and the commercialization of her cells without their knowledge or any financial compensation. In clinical settings, patients must be fully informed about what their genetic testing entails, how their data will be used, and who will have access to it.

Consent is another critical issue, especially in the context of how informed that consent is. Patients must fully understand what their genetic data will be used for, including potential future research. The case of the Havasupai tribe in Arizona, where genetic samples collected for diabetes research were later used for other studies without the tribe's informed consent, highlights the importance of clear and comprehensive consent processes.[100]

The Genetic Information Nondiscrimination Act (GINA) of 2008 in the United States is an example of legislative action taken to protect individuals' genetic privacy. GINA prevents discrimination from health insurers and employers based on genetic information, but it does not cover life, disability, or long-term care insurance, which remains a concern.[101]

Genetic discrimination occurs when individuals are treated unfairly because of differences in their DNA that may affect their health. This issue is particularly pertinent in the context of employment and insurance. For example, an individual might be denied insurance coverage or charged higher rates based on a genetic predisposition to a certain disease, even if they are currently healthy.

The fear of genetic discrimination can deter individuals from undergoing potentially life-saving genetic testing or participating in genetic research, which can have broader implications for public health and scientific advancement. While GINA in the United States is a step toward addressing this issue, gaps remain, particularly in areas not covered by the act. Moreover, there are concerns about the enforcement of such protections and the public's awareness of their rights under these laws.[102] While GINA offers some protections, its limitations highlight the need for more comprehensive policies to prevent genetic discrimination in various aspects of life.

In the healthcare sector, ethical guidelines and policies must be continually updated to keep pace with advancements in genomics. This includes ensuring that healthcare providers are trained in ethical considerations and that patients are adequately informed about the implications of genomic testing.

Legal Considerations in Genomics in Clinical Medicine

Regulatory Frameworks

The integration of genomics into clinical medicine is governed by various regulatory frameworks designed to ensure the safe, ethical, and effective use of genetic information and technologies. These frameworks address issues ranging from the approval and use of genetic tests to data privacy and intellectual property rights.

In the United States, the Food and Drug Administration (FDA) plays a key role in regulating genetic tests, ensuring their safety and effectiveness. The FDA's oversight extends to the accuracy of test results and the validity of the claims made by test manufacturers. For example, in 2013, the FDA issued a warning letter to the genetic testing company 23 and Me, instructing it to discontinue marketing its Personal Genome Service until it received FDA authorization.[103,104]

Another important regulatory aspect is the protection of genetic data. The Health Insurance Portability and Accountability Act (HIPAA) in the United States sets standards for protecting sensitive patient health information, including genetic data. Additionally, the GINA of 2008, as noted above, protects individuals from genetic discrimination in health insurance and employment, addressing concerns that genetic information could be used unfairly against individuals.

Patient Rights and Protections

Patient rights and protections are central to the ethical application of genomics in clinical medicine. These rights include informed consent, the right to privacy, and the right to access or refuse genetic testing.

Informed consent is particularly crucial in genomics, where patients must understand the potential implications of genetic testing. This includes the possible outcomes, risks, and the nature of the information that might be revealed. For instance, patients should be informed about the possibility of uncovering predispositions to certain diseases, which could have psychological and social implications.

The right to privacy is another critical aspect, ensuring that genetic information is protected and shared only with the patient's consent. This is particularly important given the sensitive nature of genetic data, which can reveal information not just about the individual but also about their family members.

Finally, patients have the right to access genetic testing and counseling services, as well as the right to refuse these services. This empowers patients to make informed decisions about their healthcare based on their values and circumstances.

Social Implications in Genomics in Clinical Medicine

Public Perception and Education

The public's perception of genomics and its role in clinical medicine significantly influences the acceptance and utilization of genomic technologies. Misconceptions and lack of understanding about genomics can lead to skepticism and apprehension toward genetic testing and personalized medicine. While there are genetic counselors who are trained to interpret results and provide education to patients to help them make informed healthcare decisions, many people are unlikely to utilize genetic counselors and opt to interpret their results on their own or see a physician instead.[105] Unfortunately, many healthcare professionals report being unprepared to answer patient questions about their patient's genomic profile.[106,107] Therefore, public education is crucial in demystifying genomics and conveying its potential benefits and limitations.[108]

Educational initiatives should aim to enhance understanding of what genomics is, how genetic testing works, and what information it can provide. This includes addressing common concerns about privacy, the meaning of genetic results, and potential implications for health insurance and employment. For example, programs such as the National Human Genome Research Institute's (NHGRI) "Genomics and Me" provide resources to educate the public about genomics.[109]

Impact on Healthcare Equity

The integration of genomics into clinical medicine also raises important questions about healthcare equity. There is a concern that advanced genomic technologies might widen existing health disparities if they are more accessible to affluent or certain demographic groups. This disparity can occur due to differences in healthcare access, affordability of genetic testing, and varying levels of genomic literacy.

For instance, studies have shown that minority populations in the United States are underrepresented in genomic research, which can lead to inequities in the benefits derived from genomic medicine.[110] Addressing these disparities requires concerted efforts to ensure that genomic medicine benefits all populations, including policies to improve access to genomic testing and treatment across different socioeconomic and ethnic groups and ensuring diversity in genomic research.

Efforts to promote healthcare equity in genomics also involve training healthcare providers to recognize and address these disparities. This includes understanding the social determinants of health that may affect a patient's access to genomic medicine and tailoring healthcare delivery to meet the diverse needs of different populations.

Conclusion

This chapter has explored the significant role of genomics in personalized medicine, highlighting its impact on therapy selection, the prevention of adverse reactions, and the tailoring of treatments for improved patient outcomes. We discussed the ethical, legal, and social implications of genomic medicine, emphasizing the importance of privacy, consent, and addressing healthcare disparities.

Looking ahead, genomic medicine is poised to become even more integral in healthcare. Advances in technology and research are expected to enhance our understanding of genetic influences on diseases, leading to more precise diagnostic tools and effective treatments. The continued integration of genomics into clinical practice promises to usher in an era of truly personalized medicine, with treatments tailored to individual genetic profiles.

For healthcare providers, staying abreast of developments in genomic medicine is crucial. As the field evolves, healthcare providers will play a pivotal role in interpreting genomic data, guiding patients through the complexities of genetic information, and integrating this knowledge into patient care. Embracing these changes will require ongoing education and adaptation, ensuring that physicians remain at the forefront of this transformative era in healthcare. Ultimately, the integration of genomics into medicine holds the promise of more informed, effective, and personalized patient care.

References

1. Lander ES, Linton LM, Birren B, Nusbaum C, Zody MC, Baldwin J, et al. International human genome sequencing consortium. Initial sequencing and analysis of the human genome. *Nature*. 2001 Feb 15;409(6822):860–921. doi:10.1038/35057062. Erratum in: *Nature*. 2001 Aug 2;412(6846):565. Erratum in: *Nature*. 2001 Jun 7;411(6838):720. Szustakowki, J [corrected to Szustakowski, J]. PMID: 11237011.
2. Shendure J, Balasubramanian S, Church G, Gilbert W, Rogers J, Schloss JA, et al. DNA sequencing at 40: past, present and future. *Nature*. 2017;550:345–353. doi:10.1038/nature24286.
3. Shastry BS. SNPs: impact on gene function and phenotype. *Methods Mol Biol*. 2009;578:3–22. doi:10.1007/978-1-60327-411-1_1. PMID: 19768584.
4. National Human Genome Research Institute. Gene Expression. NIH. 2024. https://www.genome.gov/genetics-glossary/Gene-Expression#:~:text=Definition&text=Gene%20expression%20is%20the%20process,molecules%20that%20serve%20other%20functions. Accessed 2024 Jan 8.
5. Office of Science. DOE Explains...Genomics. ENERGY.GOV. https://www.energy.gov/science/doe-explainsgenomics#:~:text=A%20genome%20is%20an%20organism's,and%20their%20roles%20in%20inheritance. Accessed 2024 Jan 8.
6. Wang Y, Chiu JF, He QY. Chapter 20 — genomics and proteomics in drug design and discovery. In: Hacker M, Messer W, Bachmann B, editors. *Pharmacology*. London: Academic Press; 2009. p. 561–573, ISBN 9780123695215. doi:10.1016/B978-0-12-369521-5.00020-8. https://www.sciencedirect.com/science/article/pii/B9780123695215000208.

7. Schultz RM. Proteins and Protein Structure☆, *Reference Module in Life Sciences*. Elsevier; 2017, ISBN 9780128096338. doi:10.1016/B978-0-12-809633-8.06969-7.

8. Bunnik EM, Le Roch KG. An introduction to functional genomics and systems biology. *Adv Wound Care (New Rochelle)*. 2013 Nov;2(9): 490–498. doi:10.1089/wound.2012.0379. PMID: 24527360; PMCID: PMC3816999.

9. Weinshilboum RM, Wang L. Pharmacogenomics: precision medicine and drug response. *Mayo Clin Proc*. 2017 Nov;92(11):1711–1722. doi:10.1016/j.mayocp.2017.09.001. Epub 2017 Nov 1. PMID: 29101939; PMCID: PMC5682947.

10. National Center for Biotechnology Information (NCBI). One Size Does Not Fit All: The Promise of Pharacogenomics. 2011. www.ncbi.nlm.nih.gov/About/primer/pharm.html. Accessed 2011 Feb 12.

11. Crews KR, Hicks JK, Pui CH, Relling MV, Evans WE. Pharmacogenomics and individualized medicine: translating science into practice. *Clin Pharmacol Ther*. 2012 Oct;92(4):467–475. doi:10.1038/clpt.2012.120. Epub 2012 Sep 5. PMID: 22948889; PMCID: PMC3589526.

12. Sivashankari S, Shanmughavel P. Comparative genomics — a perspective. *Bioinformation*. 2007 Mar 27;1(9):376–378. doi:10.6026/97320630001376. PMID: 17597925; PMCID: PMC1891719.

13. Comparative Genomics Fact Sheet. NIH. 2020. https://www.genome.gov/about-genomics/fact-sheets/Comparative-Genomics-Fact-Sheet#:~:text=Comparative%20genomics%20is%20a%20field,regions%20of%20similarity%20and%20difference. Accessed 2024 Jan 8.

14. Russell PJ. *iGenetics: A Molecular Approach*. 3rd ed. San Francisco: Pearson Benjamin Cummings; 2010. p. 217. ISBN 978-0-321-56976-9.

15. Bonetta L. Epigenomics: the new tool in studying complex diseases. *Nat Educ*. 2008;1(1):178. https://www.nature.com/scitable/topicpage/epigenomics-the-new-tool-in-studying-complex-694/. Accessed 2024 Jan 8.

16. Watson J, Crick F. Molecular structure of nucleic acids: a structure for deoxyribose nucleic acid. *Nature*. 1953;171:737–738. doi:10.1038/171737a0.

17. International Human Genome Sequencing Consortium. Finishing the euchromatic sequence of the human genome. *Nature*. 2004;431:931–945. doi:10.1038/nature03001.

18. Mardis ER. Next-generation DNA sequencing methods. *Annu Rev Genomics Hum Genet*. 2008;9:387–402. doi:10.1146/annurev.genom.9.081307.164359. PMID: 18576944.

19. Sanger F, Nicklen S, Coulson AR. DNA sequencing with chain-terminating inhibitors. *Proc Natl Acad Sci U S A.* 1977;74:5463–5467.
20. Heather JM, Chain B. The sequence of sequencers: the history of sequencing DNA. *Genomics.* 2016;107(1):1–8. doi:10.1016/j.ygeno.2015.11.003. Epub 2015 Nov 10. PMID: 26554401; PMCID: PMC4727787.
21. Korf BR. Integration of genomics into medical practice. *Discov Med.* 2013 Nov;16(89):241–248. PMID: 24229741.
22. Slamon DJ, Leyland-Jones B, Shak S, Fuchs H, Paton V, Bajamonde A, et al. Use of chemotherapy plus a monoclonal antibody against HER2 for metastatic breast cancer that overexpresses HER2. *N Engl J Med.* 2001 Mar 15;344(11):783–792. doi:10.1056/NEJM200103153441101. PMID: 11248153.
23. Relling MV, Gardner EE, Sandborn WJ, Schmiegelow K, Pui CH, Yee SW, et al. Clinical pharmacogenetics implementation consortium guidelines for thiopurine methyltransferase genotype and thiopurine dosing: 2013 update. *Clin Pharmacol Ther.* 2013 Apr;93(4):324–325. doi:10.1038/clpt.2013.4. Epub 2013 Jan 17. PMID: 23422873; PMCID: PMC3604643.
24. Bonomi L, Huang Y, Ohno-Machado L. Privacy challenges and research opportunities for genomic data sharing. *Nat Genet.* 2020 Jul;52(7):646–654. doi:10.1038/s41588-020-0651-0. Epub 2020 Jun 29. PMID: 32601475; PMCID: PMC7761157.
25. Kho A, Rasmussen L, Connolly J, Peissig PL, Starren J, Hakonarson H, et al. Practical challenges in integrating genomic data into the electronic health record. *Genet Med.* 2013;15:772–778. doi:10.1038/gim.2013.131.
26. Roberts JS, Ostergren J. Direct-to-consumer genetic testing and personal genomics services: a review of recent empirical studies. *Curr Genet Med Rep.* 2013;1:182–200. doi:10.1007/s40142-013-0018-2.
27. Evans BJ. HIPAA's individual right of access to genomic data: reconciling safety and civil rights. *Am J Hum Genet.* 2018;102:5–10. doi:10.1016/j.ajhg.2017.12.004
28. Wade CH. What is the psychosocial impact of providing genetic and genomic health information to individuals? An overview of systematic reviews. *Hastings Cent Rep.* 2019;49(Suppl. 1):S88–S96. doi:10.1002/hast.1021.
29. Mathaiyan J, Chandrasekaran A, Davis S. Ethics of genomic research. *Perspect Clin Res.* 2013 Jan;4(1):100–104. doi:10.4103/2229-3485.106405. PMID: 23533991; PMCID: PMC3601693.

30. Trinidad SB, Fryer-Edwards K, Crest A, Kyler P, Lloyd-Puryear MA, Burke W. Educational needs in genetic medicine: primary care perspectives. *Commun Genet.* 2008;11:160–165. doi:10.1159/000113878.

31. Avard, D, Knoppers, BM. Genomic medicine: considerations for health professionals and the public. *Genome Med.* 2009;1:25. doi:10.1186/gm25.

32. Caulfield T, McGuire AL, Cho M, Buchanan JA, Burgess MM, Danilczyk U, et al. Research ethics recommendations for whole-genome research: consensus statement. *PLoS Biol.* 2008;6:e73. doi:10.1371/journal.pbio. 0060073.

33. Green R, Berg J, Grody W, Kalia SS, Korf BR, Martin CL, et al. ACMG recommendations for reporting of incidental findings in clinical exome and genome sequencing. *Genet Med.* 2013;15:565–574. doi:10.1038/gim. 2013.73.

34. Weinshilboum R. Inheritance and drug response. *N Engl J Med.* 2003;348:529–537.

35. Evans WE, Relling MV. Pharmacogenomics: translating functional genomics into rational therapeutics. *Science.* 1999;286:487–491.

36. Kirchheiner J, Nickchen K, Bauer M, Wong ML, Licinio J, Roots I, et al. Pharmacogenetics of antidepressants and antipsychotics: the contribution of allelic variations to the phenotype of drug response. *Mol Psychiatry.* 2004 May;9(5):442–473. doi:10.1038/sj.mp.4001494. PMID: 15037866.

37. Mallal S, Phillips E, Carosi G, Molina JM, Workman C, Tomazic J, et al. HLA-B*5701 screening for hypersensitivity to abacavir. *N Engl J Med.* 2008 Feb 7;358(6):568–579. doi:10.1056/NEJMoa0706135. PMID: 18256392.

38. Johnson JA, Gong L, Whirl-Carrillo M, Gage BF, Scott SA, Stein CM, et al. Clinical pharmacogenetics implementation consortium guidelines for CYP2C9 and VKORC1 genotypes and warfarin dosing. *Clin Pharmacol Ther.* 2011 Oct;90(4):625–629. doi:10.1038/clpt.2011.185. Epub 2011 Sep 7. PMID: 21900891; PMCID: PMC3187550.

39. Marsh S, van Rooij T. Challenges of incorporating pharmacogenomics into clinical practice. *Gastrointest Cancer Res.* 2009 Sep;3(5):206–207. PMID: 20084163; PMCID: PMC2806804.

40. Collins FS, Varmus H. A new initiative on precision medicine. *N Engl J Med.* 2015 Feb 26;372(9):793–795. doi:10.1056/NEJMp1500523. Epub 2015 Jan 30. PMID: 25635347; PMCID: PMC5101938.

41. King MC, Marks JH, Mandell JB, New York Breast Cancer Study Group. Breast and ovarian cancer risks due to inherited mutations in BRCA1 and

BRCA2. *Science*. 2003 Oct 24;302(5645):643–646. doi:10.1126/science.1088759. PMID: 14576434.

42. Relling MV, Gardner EE, Sandborn WJ, Schmiegelow K, Pui CH, Yee SW, et al. Clinical pharmacogenetics implementation consortium guidelines for thiopurine methyltransferase genotype and thiopurine dosing. *Clin Pharmacol Ther*. 2011 Mar;89(3):387–391. doi:10.1038/clpt.2010.320. Epub 2011 Jan 26. Erratum in: *Clin Pharmacol Ther*. 2011 Dec;90(6):894. PMID: 21270794; PMCID: PMC3098761.

43. Biesecker LG, Green RC. Diagnostic clinical genome and exome sequencing. *N Engl J Med*. 2014 Jun 19;370(25):2418–2425. doi:10.1056/NEJMra1312543. PMID: 24941179.

44. Choi M, Scholl UI, Ji W, Liu T, Tikhonova IR, Zumbo P, et al. Genetic diagnosis by whole exome capture and massively parallel DNA sequencing. *Proc Natl Acad Sci U S A*. 2009 Nov 10;106(45):19096–19101. doi:10.1073/pnas.0910672106. Epub 2009 Oct 27. PMID: 19861545; PMCID: PMC2768590.

45. Cooper DN, Krawczak M, Antonorakis SE. The nature and mechanisms of human gene mutation. In: Scriver CR, Beaudet AL, Sly WS, Valle D, editors. *The Metabolic and Molecular Bases of Inherited Disease*. 7th ed. New York: McGraw-Hill; 1995. p. 259–291.

46. Topol EJ. High-performance medicine: the convergence of human and artificial intelligence. *Nat Med*. 2019;25:44–56. doi:10.1038/s41591-018-0300-7.

47. Sandford E, Burmeister M. Genes and genetic testing in hereditary ataxias. *Genes (Basel)*. 2014;15:586–603.

48. Sun M, Johnson AK, Nelakuditi V, Guidugli L, Fischer D, Arndt K, et al. Targeted exome analysis identifies the genetic basis of disease in over 50% of patients with a wide range of ataxia-related phenotypes. *Genet Med*. 2019 Jan;21(1):195–206. doi:10.1038/s41436-018-0007-7. Epub 2018 Jun 18. PMID: 29915382; PMCID: PMC6524765.

49. Németh AH, Kwasniewska AC, Lise S, Parolin Schnekenberg R, Becker EB, Bera KD, et al. Next generation sequencing for molecular diagnosis of neurological disorders using ataxias as a model. *Brain*. 2013 Oct;136(Pt 10):3106–3118. doi:10.1093/brain/awt236. Epub 2013 Sep 11. PMID: 24030952; PMCID: PMC3784284.

50. Bhullar KS, Lagarón NO, McGowan EM, Parmar I, Jha A, Hubbard BP, et al. Kinase-targeted cancer therapies: progress, challenges and future directions. *Mol Cancer*. 2018;17(1):48.

51. Krzyszczyk P, Acevedo A, Davidoff EJ, Timmins LM, Marrero-Berrios I, Patel M, et al. The growing role of precision and personalized medicine for cancer treatment. *Technology (Singap World Sci).* 2018 Sep-Dec;6(3–4):79–100. doi:10.1142/S2339547818300020. Epub 2019 Jan 11. PMID: 30713991; PMCID: PMC6352312.

52. Strausberg RL, Simpson AJG, Old LJ, Riggins GJ. Oncogenomics and the development of new cancer therapies. *Nature.* 2004;429(6990):469–474.

53. Grewal JK, Tessier-Cloutier B, Jones M, Gakkhar S, Ma Y, Moore R, et al. Application of a neural network whole transcriptome-based pan-cancer method for diagnosis of primary and metastatic cancers. *JAMA Netw Open.* 2019;2:e192597.

54. Penson A, Camacho N, Zheng Y, Varghese AM, Al-Ahmadie H, Razavi P, et al. Development of genome-derived tumor type prediction to inform clinical cancer care. *JAMA Oncol.* 2019;6:84–91.

55. Ohashi K, Sequist LV, Arcila ME, Moran T, Chmielecki J, Lin YL, et al. Lung cancers with acquired resistance to EGFR inhibitors occasionally harbor BRAF gene mutations but lack mutations in KRAS, NRAS, or MEK1. *Proc Natl Acad Sci U S A.* 2012;109:E2127–E2133. doi:10.1073/pnas.1203530109.

56. Koivunen JP, Mermel C, Zejnullahu K, Murphy C, Lifshits E, Holmes AJ, et al. EML4-ALK fusion gene and efficacy of an ALK kinase inhibitor in lung cancer. *Clin Cancer Res.* 2008;14:4275–4283. doi:10.1158/1078-0432.CCR-08-0168.

57. Kikuchi T, Daigo Y, Katagiri T, Tsunoda T, Okada K, Kakiuchi S, et al. Expression profiles of non-small cell lung cancers on cDNA microarrays: identification of genes for prediction of lymph-node metastasis and sensitivity to anti-cancer drugs. *Oncogene.* 2003;22:2192–2205. doi:10.1038/sj.onc.1206288.

58. Podolsky MD, Barchuk AA, Kuznetcov VI, Gusarova NF, Gaidukov VS, Tarakanov SA. Evaluation of machine learning algorithm utilization for lung cancer classification based on gene expression levels. *Asian Pac J Cancer Prev.* 2016;17:835–838. doi:10.7314/APJCP.2016.17.2.835.

59. Rizvi NA, Hellmann MD, Snyder A, Kvistborg P, Makarov V, Havel JJ, et al. Mutational landscape determines sensitivity to PD-1 blockade in non-small cell lung cancer. *Science.* 2015 Apr 3;348(6230):124–128. doi:10.1126/science.aaa1348. Epub 2015 Mar 12. PMID: 25765070; PMCID: PMC4993154.

60. Kuchenbaecker KB, Hopper JL, Barnes DR, Phillips KA, Mooij TM, Roos-Blom MJ, et al. Risks of breast, ovarian, and contralateral breast cancer for BRCA1 and BRCA2 mutation carriers. *JAMA*. 2017 Jun 20;317(23):2402–2416. doi:10.1001/jama.2017.7112. PMID: 28632866.

61. MacDonald ME, Ambrose CM, Duyao MP, Myers RH, Lin C, Srinidhi L, et al. A novel gene containing a trinucleotide repeat that is expanded and unstable on Huntington's disease chromosomes. *Cell*. 1993 Mar 26;72(6):971–983. doi:10.1016/0092-8674(93)90585-e. PMID: 8458085.

62. Pagon RA, Hanson NB, Neufeld-Kaiser W, Covington ML. Genetic testing. *West J Med*. 2001 May;174(5):344–347. doi:10.1136/ewjm.174.5.344. PMID: 11342518; PMCID: PMC1071396.

63. Spear BB, Heath-Chiozzi M, Huff J. Clinical application of pharmacogenetics. *Trends Mol Med*. 2001;7:201–204.

64. Aneesh TP, Sekhar S, Jose A, Chandran L, Zachariah SM. Pharmacogenomics: the right drug to the right person. *J Clin Med Res*. 2009 Oct;1(4):191–194. doi:10.4021/jocmr2009.08.1255. Epub 2009 Oct 16. PMID: 22461867; PMCID: PMC3299179.

65. Kalow W, Tang BK, Endrenyi L. Hypothesis: comparisons of inter- and intra-individual variations can substitute for twin studies in drug research. *Pharmacogenetics*. 1998;8:283–289.

66. Reuter JA, Spacek DV, Snyder MP. High-throughput sequencing technologies. *Mol Cell*. 2015 May 21;58(4):586–597. doi:10.1016/j.molcel.2015.05.004. PMID: 26000844; PMCID: PMC4494749.

67. Grumbt B, Eck SH, Hinrichsen T, Hirv K. Diagnostic applications of next generation sequencing in immunogenetics and molecular oncology. *Transfus Med Hemother*. 2013;40: 196–206. doi:10.1159/000351267.

68. Vrijenhoek T, Kraaijeveld K, Elferink M, de Ligt J, Kranen-donk E, Santen G, et al. Next-generation sequencing-based genome diagnostics across clinical genetics centers: implementation choices and their effects. *Eur J Hum Genet*. 2015;23:1142–1150. doi:10.1038/ejhg.2014.279.

69. Koboldt DC, Steinberg KM, Larson DE, Wilson RK, Mardis ER. The next-generation sequencing revolution and its impact on genomics. *Cell*. 2013 Sep 26;155(1):27–38. doi:10.1016/j.cell.2013.09.006. PMID: 24074859; PMCID: PMC3969849.

70. Thorburn F, Bennett S, Modha S, Murdoch D, Gunson R, Murcia PR. The use of next generation sequencing in the diagnosis and typing of respiratory infections. *J Clin Virol*. 2015;69:96–100. doi:10.1016/j.jcv.2015.06.082.

71. Gorokhova S, Biancalana V, Lévy N, Laporte J, Bartoli M, Krahn M. Clinical massively parallel sequencing for the diagnosis of myopathies. *Rev Neurol (Paris)*. 2015;171:558–571. doi:10.1016/j.neurol.2015.02.019.

72. Rehm HL. Disease-targeted sequencing: a cornerstone in the clinic. *Nat Rev Genet*. 2013 Apr;14(4):295–300. doi:10.1038/nrg3463. Epub 2013 Mar 12. PMID: 23478348; PMCID: PMC3786217.

73. Peters DG, Yatsenko SA, Surti U, Rajkovic A. Recent advances of genomic testing in perinatal medicine. *Semin Perinatol*. 2015;39:44–54. doi:10.1053/j.semperi.2014.10.009.

74. Jennings LJ, Arcila ME, Corless C, Kamel-Reid S, Lubin IM, Pfeifer J, et al. Guidelines for validation of next-generation sequencing-based oncology panels: a joint consensus recommendation of the Association for Molecular Pathology and College of American Pathologists. *J Mol Diagn*. 2017 May;19(3):341–365. doi:10.1016/j.jmoldx.2017.01.011. Epub 2017 Mar 21. PMID: 28341590; PMCID: PMC6941185.

75. Jamuar SS, Tan EC. Clinical application of next-generation sequencing for Mendelian diseases. *Hum Genomics*. 2015;9:10. doi:10.1186/s40246-015-0031-5.

76. Carrera P, Di Resta C, Volonteri C, Castiglioni E, Bonfiglio S, Lazarevic D, et al. Exome sequencing and pathway analysis for identification of genetic variability relevant for bronchopulmonary dysplasia (BPD) in preterm newborns: a pilot study. *Clin Chim Acta*. 2015;451:39–45. doi:10.1016/j.cca.2015.01.001.

77. Di Resta C, Spiga I, Presi S, Merella S, Pipitone GB, Manitto MP, et al. Integration of multigene panels for the diagnosis of hereditary retinal disorders using next generation sequencing and bioinformatics approaches. *EJIFCC*. 2018;29:15–25.

78. Doyle MA, Li J, Doig K, Fellowes A, Wong SQ. Studying cancer genomics through next-generation DNA sequencing and bioinformatics. *Methods Mol Biol*. 2014;1168:83–98. doi:10.1007/978-1-4939-0847-9_6.

79. Pereira R, Oliveira J, Sousa M. Bioinformatics and computational tools for next-generation sequencing analysis in clinical genetics. *J Clin Med*. 2020 Jan 3;9(1):132. doi:10.3390/jcm9010132. PMID: 31947757; PMCID: PMC7019349.

80. Peake I. The polymerase chain reaction. *J Clin Pathol*. 1989 Jul;42(7):673–676. doi:10.1136/jcp.42.7.673. PMID: 2668341; PMCID: PMC1142012.

81. Saiki RK, Gelfand DH, Stoffel S, Scharf SJ, Higuchi R, Horn GT, et al. Primer-directed enzymatic amplification of DNA with a thermostable DNA

polymerase. *Science*. 1988 Jan 29;239(4839):487–491. doi:10.1126/science.2448875. PMID: 2448875.

82. Boehm CD. Use of polymerase chain reaction for diagnosis of inherited disorders. *Clin Chem*. 1989 Sep;35(9):1843–1848. PMID: 2570652.

83. Qin D. Next-generation sequencing and its clinical application. *Cancer Biol Med*. 2019 Feb;16(1):4–10. doi:10.20892/j.issn.2095-3941.2018.0055. PMID: 31119042; PMCID: PMC6528456.

84. Schena M, Shalon D, Davis RW, Brown PO. Quantitative monitoring of gene expression patterns with a complementary DNA microarray. *Science*. 1995 Oct 20;270(5235):467–470. doi:10.1126/science.270.5235.467. PMID: 7569999.

85. Relling MV, Evans WE. Pharmacogenomics in the clinic. *Nature*. 2015;7573:343–350.

86. Relling MV, Klein TE. CPIC: Clinical pharmacogenetics implementation consortium of the pharmacogenomics research network. *Clin Pharmacol Ther*. 2011;3:464–467.

87. Brown SA, Pereira N. Pharmacogenomic impact of CYP2C19 variation on clopidogrel therapy in precision cardiovascular medicine. *J Pers Med*. 2018 Jan 30;8(1):8. doi:10.3390/jpm8010008. PMID: 29385765; PMCID: PMC5872082.

88. Dean L. Warfarin therapy and VKORC1 and CYP genotype. 2012 Mar 8 [Updated 2018 Jun 11]. In: Pratt VM, Scott SA, Pirmohamed M, Esquivel B, Kattman BL, Malheiro AJ, editors. *Medical Genetics Summaries* [Internet]. Bethesda: National Center for Biotechnology Information (US); 2012. https://www.ncbi.nlm.nih.gov/books/NBK84174/.

89. Floyd JS, Psaty BM. The application of genomics in diabetes: barriers to discovery and implementation. *Diabetes Care*. 2016 Nov;39(11):1858–1869. doi:10.2337/dc16-0738. PMID: 27926887; PMCID: PMC5079615.

90. Francke U, Dijamco C, Kiefer AK, Eriksson N, Moiseff B, Tung JY, et al. Dealing with the unexpected: consumer responses to direct-access BRCA mutation testing. *Peer J*. 2013;1:e8. doi:10.7717/peerj.8.

91. Strianese O, Rizzo F, Ciccarelli M, Galasso G, D'Agostino Y, Salvati A, et al. Precision and personalized medicine: how genomic approach improves the management of cardiovascular and neurodegenerative disease. *Genes (Basel)*. 2020 Jul 6;11(7):747. doi:10.3390/genes11070747. PMID: 32640513; PMCID: PMC7397223.

92. Micaglio E, Locati ET, Monasky MM, Romani F, Heilbron F, Pappone C. Role of pharmacogenetics in adverse drug reactions: an update towards

personalized medicine. *Front Pharmacol.* 2021 Apr 30;12:651720. doi:10.3389/fphar.2021.651720. PMID: 33995067; PMCID: PMC8120428.

93. Lazarou J. Pomeranz BH. Corey PN. Incidence of adverse drug reactions in hospitalized patients: a meta-analysis of prospective studies. *JAMA.* 1998;279:1200–1205.

94. Coleman JJ, Pontefract SK. Adverse drug reactions. *Clin Med (Lond).* 2016 Oct;16(5):481–485. doi:10.7861/clinmedicine.16-5-481. PMID: 27697815; PMCID: PMC6297296.

95. Dean L. Abacavir therapy and HLA-B*57:01 genotype. 2015 Sep 1 [Updated 2018 Apr 18]. In: Pratt VM, Scott SA, Pirmohamed M, Esquivel B, Kattman BL, Malheiro AJ, editors. *Medical Genetics Summaries* [Internet]. Bethesda: National Center for Biotechnology Information (US); 2012. https://www.ncbi.nlm.nih.gov/books/NBK315783/.

96. Hippman C, Nislow C. Pharmacogenomic testing: clinical evidence and implementation challenges. *J Pers Med.* 2019 Aug 7;9(3):40. doi:10.3390/jpm9030040. PMID: 31394823; PMCID: PMC6789586.

97. Slamon D, Eiermann W, Robert N, Pienkowski T, Martin M, Press M, et al. Adjuvant trastuzumab in HER2-positive breast cancer. *N Engl J Med.* 2011;365(14):1273–1283.

98. Ramsey BW, Davies J, McElvaney NG, Tullis E, Bell SC, Dřevínek P, et al. A CFTR potentiator in patients with cystic fibrosis and the G551D mutation. *N Engl J Med.* 2011 Nov 3;365(18):1663–1672. doi:10.1056/NEJMoa1105185. PMID: 22047557; PMCID: PMC3230303.

99. Skloot R. *The Immortal Life of Henrietta Lacks.* New York: Crown; 2010. ASIN: 1400052181.

100. Mello MM, Wolf LE. The Havasupai Indian tribe case--lessons for research involving stored biologic samples. *N Engl J Med.* 2010 Jul 15;363(3):204–207. doi:10.1056/NEJMp1005203. Epub 2010 Jun 9. PMID: 20538622.

101. Hudson KL, Holohan MK, Collins FS. Keeping pace with the times — the genetic information nondiscrimination act of 2008. *N Engl J Med.* 2008 June 19;358:2661–2663. doi:10.1056/NEJMp0803964.

102. Rothstein MA. Currents in contemporary ethics. GINA, the ADA, and genetic discrimination in employment. *J Law Med Ethics.* 2008 Winter;36(4):837–840. doi:10.1111/j.1748-720X.2008.00341.x. PMID: 19094010; PMCID: PMC3035561.

103. 23andMe and the FDA. 23andMe. https://customercare.23andme.com/hc/en-us/articles/211831908-23andMe-and-the-FDA#:~:text=In%20 2013%2C%2023andMe%20received%20a,the%20agency's%20regulatory%20review%20process.

104. Zhang S. 23andMe ordered to halt sales of DNA tests. *Nature.* 2013. doi:10.1038/nature.2013.14236.

105. Markens S. 'I'm not sure if they speak to everyone about this option': analyzing disparate access to and use of genetic health services in the US from the perspective of genetic counselors. *Crit Public Health.* 2017;27:111–124. doi:10.1080/09581596.2016.1179263.

106. Schaibley VM, Ramos IN, Woosley RL, Curry S, Hays S, Ramos KS. Limited genomics training among physicians remains a barrier to genomics-based implementation of precision medicine. *Front Med (Lausanne).* 2022 Mar 18;9:757212. doi:10.3389/fmed.2022.757212. PMID: 35372454; PMCID: PMC8971187.

107. Desmond A, Kurian AW, Gabree M, Mills MA, Anderson MJ, Kobayashi Y, et al. Clinical actionability of multigene panel testing for hereditary breast and ovarian cancer risk assessment. *JAMA Oncol.* 2015;1:943–951. doi:10.1001/jamaoncol.2015.2690.

107. Tuttle TM, Jarosek S, Habermann EB, Arrington A, Abraham A, Morris TJ, et al. Increasing rates of contralateral prophylactic mastectomy among patients with ductal carcinoma in situ. *J Clin Oncol.* 2009;27:1362–1367. doi:10.1200/JCO.2008.20.1681.

108. Whitley KV, Tueller JA, Weber KS. Genomics education in the era of personal genomics: academic, professional, and public considerations. *Int J Mol Sci.* 2020 Jan 24;21(3):768. doi:10.3390/ijms21030768. PMID: 31991576; PMCID: PMC7037382.

109. National Human Genome Research Institute. https://www.genome.gov/. Accessed 2024 Jan 16.

110. Popejoy A, Fullerton S. Genomics is failing on diversity. *Nature.* 2016;538:161–164. doi:10.1038/538161a.

Chapter 6

Organ-on-a-Chip: Revolutionizing Medical Research

Introduction

The process of developing new drugs is notably time consuming and costly. It typically takes 10–15 years to bring a new drug to market, with an average expenditure of around $5 billion.[1] Breaking down these costs, preclinical development is responsible for 63% of the total, while clinical trials comprise 32% of the expenditure.[2] A significant challenge in this process is the reliance on animal models and cell lines derived from animals during the preclinical phase. This reliance is problematic due to the significant biological differences between species, particularly in ion channels, metabolic pathways, and pharmacokinetics.[3] Indeed, numerous pharmaceuticals have advanced through preclinical and clinical stages and have been on the market — sometimes for several years — before being withdrawn by the U.S. Food and Drug Administration (FDA) due to unforeseen human toxicity. One study estimates that approximately 40% of new drugs fail in clinical trials due to unpredictable responses and unforeseen toxicity in humans despite successfully passing preclinical evaluations using animal models.[4] A key factor contributing to this unsuccessful transition from promising drug candidates to safe, widely used treatments is the absence of model systems that effectively mimic the normal functioning of human organs and their reactions to medicinal compounds.

These differences mean that animal models often do not accurately mirror human physiology, leading to unreliable predictions of human toxicity in many instances.[5] Because of these difficulties, new techniques were sought.

Organ-on-a-chip (OOC) technology represents a transformative development in medical research, addressing the limitations of traditional drug development methods such as cell cultures and animal models. This innovative approach employs microfluidic systems to create scaled-down, functional models of human organs. These microfluidic platforms, comprising tiny chambers, channels, and sensors, are engineered to simulate human organs' intricate microarchitecture and physiological functions.

Integrating living cells and tissues into these microfabricated environments is central to OOC technology. This design allows for cultivating various cell types, including primary human cells and stem cells, in conditions that closely mirror the natural environment of actual organs.[6] By accurately replicating human organs' structural and functional aspects, OOC platforms offer enhanced precision in studying human physiology, disease modeling, drug discovery, and toxicity testing.[7]

Additionally, they facilitate detailed, real-time observation and in vitro examination of living cells' biochemical, genetic, and metabolic functions within a simulated tissue and organ environment. OOC technology's potential to revolutionize medical research and drug development lies in its ability to provide more precise and efficient ways to investigate organ function and disease mechanisms.[8]

Materials Used in OOC Construction

The construction of OOC devices primarily utilizes biocompatible and flexible materials, with polydimethylsiloxane (PDMS) being the most common. PDMS is favored for its transparency, crucial for microscopic observations, and its gas permeability, essential for cell respiration. Additionally, its flexibility allows for creating dynamic mechanical environments that mimic the physical movements of organs, such as the lung's breathing or the heart's pulsations.[9]

Techniques in Microfabrication and Microfluidics

Microfabrication techniques are central to creating OOC devices. These techniques involve soft lithography, photolithography, and 3D printing, which are used to construct the intricate network of microfluidic channels and chambers that form the basis of OOCs. Soft lithography, especially, is widely used for PDMS-based microfluidic devices due to its precision and cost-effectiveness. Soft lithography is a collection of techniques based on printing, molding, and embossing with an elastomeric stamp. Microfluidics is the science of manipulating fluids at a microscale, typically in channels with dimensions of tens to hundreds of micrometers. The fundamental characteristic of microfluidics is its ability to control and handle tiny volumes of fluids, often in the range of picoliters (10^{-12} L) to nanoliters (10^{-9} L), within microscale channels.[10] Microfluidics plays a critical role in controlling the flow of nutrients, oxygen, and drugs within the OOC, thereby simulating the body's circulatory system.

Integration of Sensors and Readout Mechanisms

Integrating sensors and readout mechanisms is a vital aspect of OOC design, enabling the real-time monitoring of cellular responses and organ functions. These sensors can measure pH, oxygen levels, and mechanical forces. Advanced OOCs incorporate microelectrodes or optical sensors for electrophysiological measurements, which are crucial in heart and brain chips. Additionally, integrating microfluidic technology with electronic readouts, known as "lab-on-a-chip," allows for automated data collection and analysis, enhancing the efficiency and accuracy of the research.

Examples of OOC Models

Lung-on-a-Chip

This chip simulates the mechanical and biological characteristics of the human lung. It has been used to model lung diseases and test drug responses. The lung-on-a-chip can replicate breathing motions and has been instrumental in studying pulmonary conditions[11] and the effects of environmental toxins. For example, researchers using this device found that cyclic mechanical strain accentuates the lung's toxic and inflammatory responses to silica nanoparticles.

Heart-on-a-Chip

This model replicates the cardiac tissue's structure and function. It is used for studying heart diseases, drug screening, and understanding the cardiac tissue's response to mechanical stress.[12]

Liver-on-a-Chip

Liver chips are designed to mimic the liver's cellular architecture and function, making them helpful in studying liver diseases, metabolism, and drug detoxification processes.[13]

Brain-on-a-Chip

This chip models the neural networks and can be used to study brain physiology, neurodegenerative diseases, and the effects of drugs on the brain.

Gut-on-a-Chip

This model replicates the intestinal microenvironment and is used to study gut physiology, microbiome interactions, and intestinal diseases.[14]

Historical Context and Development

The roots of OOC can be traced back to the early 2000s. Researchers sought to move beyond the constraints of 2D cell cultures that failed to accurately represent the cellular microenvironments found in vivo. The evolution toward 3D systems culminated in the introduction of "micro-physiological systems" by Lee et al.,[15] which aimed to mimic the complexity and interactions of human tissues more faithfully. This shift has been pivotal in advancing drug testing and toxicity screening methods.

Advantages of OOC over Traditional Models

Comparison with Animal Models and 2D Cell Cultures

OOC technology offers significant advantages over traditional research models, particularly when compared to animal models and 2D cell cultures. While providing a whole-organism perspective, animal models often fail to predict human responses accurately due to interspecies differences. Additionally, ethical concerns and high costs are associated with animal research. On the other hand, 2D cell cultures, despite being a staple in biological research, lack the complex 3D structure and cell–cell interactions present in human tissues, limiting their physiological relevance.[7]

Increased Physiological Relevance

OOC systems provide a more physiologically relevant model by replicating the 3D architecture of human organs, including the specific cellular environments and mechanical forces. OOC systems permit precise control over the cellular and mechanical environment, enabling the study of drug effects under various conditions that mimic the dynamic nature of the human body. This allows for a more accurate simulation of organ functions and interactions. For instance, lung-on-a-chip models can replicate the mechanical act of breathing, which is crucial for studying respiratory diseases and treatments.[11] Similarly, by adjusting flow rates and mechanical forces in a heart-on-a-chip model, researchers can study the cardiotoxic effects of drugs under different physiological conditions.[16]

Improved Toxicity Testing

By recreating specific organs' physiological conditions and functions, OOC devices provide a more accurate representation of human biology than traditional methods such as animal testing or cell cultures. Using OOC devices, researchers can simulate the behavior of organs in a controlled laboratory setting.[17] This allows them to assess the toxicity and potential side effects of new medications more comprehensively and reliably.

By utilizing OOC technology for toxicity testing, researchers can observe how a specific organ responds to a medication in real time, mimicking the physiological conditions of the human body. This enables them to accurately assess the drug's potential toxicity and its effects on specific organs or organ systems.

Additionally, OOC devices allow for simultaneous testing of multiple organs, mimicking the interconnectedness of different organs within the body. This integrated approach helps researchers understand how different organs may interact and how potential toxicities may propagate throughout the body.

Potential for Personalized Medicine

OOC technology's potential in personalized medicine is fascinating and transformative. OOC technology can create patient-specific models using cells derived from individual patients. This aspect of OOC technology leverages the ability to use cells derived from individual patients, often through innovative techniques such as induced pluripotent stem cell (iPSC) technology. iPSCs have been genetically reprogrammed to an embryonic stem cell-like state, enabling them to differentiate into various cell types relevant to different organs. When integrated into OOC systems, these patient-specific cells can create models that closely mimic the unique physiological characteristics of an individual's organs.[18]

This personalized modeling is a significant leap forward for several reasons:

Enhanced Drug Efficacy and Safety

Traditional drug testing methods rely on average responses from large populations, which can overlook individual variations in drug metabolism and efficacy. OOC models using patient-derived cells allow for the assessment of drug responses at a personal level. This can lead to identifying the most effective drug and dosage for a specific patient, thereby increasing the likelihood of successful treatment outcomes and reducing the risk of adverse drug reactions.

Understanding Individual Variability

Different patients can respond differently to the same treatment due to genetic, environmental, and lifestyle factors. OOC technology can help understand these individual differences by providing a platform to study how specific genetic mutations or other factors influence disease progression and treatment response.

Accelerating Personalized Therapy Development

In the context of diseases with high variability among individuals, such as many cancers and genetic disorders, OOC technology can accelerate the development of personalized therapies. By testing therapeutic agents on cells that carry the patient's specific disease traits, researchers can more rapidly identify potential treatments tailored to individual needs.

Reducing Reliance on Animal Testing

Personalized OOC models can reduce the need for animal testing, which, aside from ethical considerations, often fails to accurately predict human responses due to interspecies differences. This shift aligns with ethical research practices, improves the relevance and accuracy of preclinical studies, and potentially reduces the time and costs associated with animal testing. An example is the development of lung-on-a-chip models for toxicity testing of inhaled substances that reduce the reliance on animal inhalation studies, which are often complex and expensive.[19]

Current Advances in OOC Technology

Multiorgan Integration

Recent developments in OOC technology have led to the creation of sophisticated "body-on-a-chip" or "human-on-a-chip" systems. These advanced models can simulate interactions between multiple organs, offering a comprehensive view of systemic responses to medications and diseases. This holistic approach is crucial for understanding complex human physiology.[20]

Use of Human iPSCs

There is a growing trend in employing human induced pluripotent stem cells (iPSCs) in OOC models. iPSCs are versatile and capable of differentiating into various cell types. This adaptability enables the development of patient-specific models, significantly enhancing the potential of OOCs in personalized medicine.[18]

High-Throughput Drug Screening

OOCs are increasingly designed for high-throughput screening, allowing rapid evaluation of multiple drug candidates or toxicological analyses. This capability is vital for expediting drug development and reducing associated costs.[9]

Sensor Integration and Automation

State-of-the-art OOCs now feature integrated sensors for real-time tracking of biological changes, including pH and oxygen levels. Combined with automated systems, these enhancements facilitate continuous, precise data collection and analysis, improving research efficiency and accuracy.[21,22]

Disease Modeling

The application of OOC technology in modeling complex diseases represents a significant advancement in biomedical research. This technology offers profound insights into disease mechanisms and facilitates the development of novel therapeutics.[23] Its versatility allows it to model a wide range of diseases, from cancers and neurodegenerative disorders to infectious diseases, each with unique challenges and requirements.

Cancer Research

In cancer research, OOC technology provides a dynamic platform for studying tumor growth, metastasis, and microenvironment.[24] Traditional cancer models often fail to replicate tumors' complex 3D structures and cell–cell interactions. OOC models can overcome these limitations by replicating the 3D architecture of cancer tissues, allowing for studying tumor cell behavior in a more physiologically relevant context. This includes understanding how cancer cells interact with surrounding tissues, how they respond to various anticancer drugs, and how they might develop resistance to treatments.

Neurodegenerative Disorders

Neurological disorders account for an estimated 6.3% of the global disease burden.[25] However, developing drugs for central nervous system (CNS) disorders is particularly challenging and prone to failure. The approval process for CNS drugs typically takes 38% longer compared to drugs for non-CNS conditions.[26] OOC techniques may provide a quicker, cheaper path to drug development. For neurodegenerative diseases such as Alzheimer's and Parkinson's, OOC technology offers a platform to study the intricate workings of the brain's cellular and molecular environment.[27] Brain-on-a-chip models can mimic the neural tissue's complexity, enabling researchers to study the pathophysiology of these disorders in real time. This includes analyzing the role of amyloid plaques, tau protein tangles, and other factors in neurodegeneration. Such models are invaluable for screening potential neuroprotective drugs and understanding the disease's progression at a cellular level.[28]

Infectious Diseases

Animal experiments, commonly used in developing treatments for infectious diseases, face several challenges. They often require extensive optimization over a long period, are expensive, and raise ethical issues.[29,30] Additionally, many pathogens are specific to certain species, making it hard to replicate the disease accurately in animal models. This species dependence complicates applying findings from animal studies to human cases.[31] OOC technology, which uses human cells, obviates many of these challenges.

OOC technology is also pivotal in studying infectious diseases, especially in the context of emerging pathogens and antibiotic resistance.[32] Lung-on-a-chip models, for instance, have been used to study respiratory infections, including COVID-19. These models can replicate the lung's response to pathogens, providing insights into disease progression and the efficacy of antiviral drugs. Additionally, gut-on-a-chip models study gastrointestinal infections, inflammatory bowel disease, and the microbiome's role in health and disease.[33,34]

Vascularization and Fluid Dynamics

Advanced OOCs now include features that mimic vascular structures and dynamic fluid flow, mirroring the in vivo environment more closely.[35] These features are essential for studying processes such as cancer metastasis and enhancing drug delivery research.[36]

Biomaterial Developments

Ongoing research is focused on creating new biomaterials for OOC construction. These materials aim to replicate the natural extracellular matrix more accurately, improving cell functionality and longevity within the chips.[37]

Regulatory and Ethical Focus

With the increasing prevalence of OOC technology, there is a heightened focus on regulatory and ethical considerations, especially in its application to drug testing and personalized medicine. Issues surrounding the use of human cells are being addressed with greater scrutiny.[38]

Challenges and Limitations of OOC Technology

While OOC technology offers transformative potential in biomedical research and drug development, several challenges and limitations must be addressed. This section delves into the technical and fabrication challenges and biological challenges such as cell sourcing, longevity, complexity, and regulatory and adoption hurdles.

Technical and Fabrication Challenges

Microfabrication Complexity

The intricate design of OOC systems requires advanced microscale engineering and microfabrication techniques, which can be complex and costly. Ensuring reproducibility and scalability for widespread use remains a significant challenge.[11]

Material Biocompatibility

Selecting materials that are biocompatible and can mimic the mechanical properties of the native extracellular matrix is challenging.[39] The materials must also be compatible with imaging and analytical techniques. Recent developments in biomedical engineering have led to the creation of microscale heart tissue models using microfluidic OOC systems.[40] These systems are commonly made from poly(dimethyl siloxane) (PDMS), a material chosen for its biocompatibility, nontoxic nature, and affordability.[41] Additionally, PDMS is flexible, transparent, and easily shaped into microfluidic designs through soft lithography and photolithography techniques.[42] This makes it an ideal material for rapidly producing customized OOC models.

Biological Challenges

Cell Sourcing

The emergence of iPSC technology has made obtaining patient-specific stem cells with minimal invasiveness easier.[43] iPSCs are versatile and can be transformed into different types of cells. This feature is especially beneficial for creating tissues that match a patient's human leukocyte antigen (HLA) profile in multi-organ-on-a-chip (multi-OOC) systems.[44] However, obtaining human cells that accurately represent the diversity of patient populations is a significant challenge. The use of primary cells, stem cells, or differentiated cells each comes with limited availability, variability, and ethical concerns.[45]

Longevity and Complexity

Maintaining the viability and functionality of cells in OOC systems over extended periods is challenging. Furthermore, replicating the complex interactions of human organs, including immune responses and hormonal signaling, is still a significant hurdle.[9] Maintaining cell viability and functionality over extended periods in OOC systems presents significant challenges. This difficulty is compounded when attempting to replicate the intricate interactions of human organs, such as immune responses and hormonal signaling.

Long-Term Viability and Functionality

In OOC systems, cells must survive and function effectively for extended periods to yield meaningful data. This requires a carefully controlled microenvironment, including nutrient supply, waste removal, and appropriate physical stimuli. However, over time, cells in OOC systems can experience stress or exhaustion, leading to altered functionality or cell death.

The study by Sung et al.[46] using a liver-on-a-chip model highlighted the challenges of maintaining liver cell functions over extended periods, which is crucial for long-term toxicity studies.

Complex Organ Interactions

Human organs do not function in isolation; they interact in complex ways, influenced by the immune system and hormonal signals. Replicating these interactions in OOC systems is challenging. For instance, the immune system involves dynamic interactions between various cell types and signaling molecules, which are difficult to mimic in vitro. For example, in a study by Maschmeyer et al.,[46] researchers developed a multiorgan chip integrating human skin, liver, and immune system models. Despite its success, the study highlighted the complexity of accurately replicating immune responses and organ crosstalk.[47]

Hormonal Signaling

Hormones play a critical role in regulating organ functions. In OOC systems, replicating the endocrine system's complex hormonal signaling pathways is formidable. This includes the production and secretion of hormones and their dynamic interactions with multiple organs. A study by Wagner et al. on a body-on-a-chip system attempted to incorporate hormonal signaling pathways. The research underscored the complexity of integrating endocrine functions with other organ models to achieve a holistic representation of body physiology.[48]

Regulatory and Adoption Hurdles

Standardization and Validation

For OOC technology to be widely adopted, especially in drug testing and regulatory processes, standardization of protocols and validation of models are essential. This includes demonstrating reproducibility and relevance to human physiology. Several consortia have published position papers outlining a shared vision among numerous stakeholders about the need for standardization to progress the OOC field. For instance, the ORCHID project has pinpointed standardization as a critical factor for advancing European OOC technologies.[49] Similarly, the 2019 workshop report by the Transatlantic Think Tank for Toxicology (t4) compiled insights from 46 international stakeholders,[50] and the Standards Coordinating Body in the United States is pushing for international standards for OOC platforms.

Regulatory Acceptance

Gaining acceptance from regulatory bodies such as the FDA for using OOC systems in drug approval processes is a significant challenge. Approval involves demonstrating that OOC models are as predictive, or more so, than current animal models. Before OOCs can be used, detailed and standardized protocols and reproducible results in an inter-laboratory setting are required[51] to develop a consensus.[52]

As of this writing, organs-on-a-chip (OOC) technology has yet to be formally approved by the FDA as a standalone tool for drug testing or diagnostic purposes. However, the FDA has shown interest in its potential.

The FDA has collaborated to evaluate the effectiveness of OOC systems. For instance, the FDA has collaborated with Emulate, Inc., a company specializing in OOC technology, to use their "Human Emulation System," which includes organs-on-chips, to study how human organs respond to medicines, chemicals, and diseases.[53] These collaborations aim to understand better the potential of OOC technology in improving and accelerating drug development and regulatory evaluations.

Conclusion

OOC technology, integrating microfabrication and tissue engineering, offers microfluidic devices that emulate human organ functions. This chapter highlighted its potential for more physiologically relevant drug testing and disease modeling using human and patient-specific cells. However, challenges such as long-term cell viability, complex organ inter-actions, and regulatory acceptance remain.

OOC technology is poised to transform drug development by enhancing drug screening accuracy, reducing animal testing, and aiding in personalized medicine. As technology advances, it could become a crucial tool in regulatory science, improving new therapies' safety and efficacy evaluation.

OOC technology represents a significant advancement in medical research and pharmaceutical development. Its ability to closely mimic human physiology promises to streamline drug development, offer more precise disease models, and facilitate personalized therapeutic approaches. Overcoming current challenges will be critical to its integration into mainstream research and clinical practice, potentially marking a new era in healthcare innovation.

References

1. Herper M. The Cost of Creating a New Drug Now $5 Billion, Pushing Big Pharma to Change. *Forbes*; 2013 Aug 11. http://www.forbes.com/sites/matthewherper/2013/08/11/how-the-staggering-cost-of-inventing-new-drugs-is-shaping-the-future-of-medicine/.
2. Paul SM, Mytelka DS, Dunwiddie CT, Persinger CC, Munos BH, Lindborg SR, et al. How to improve R&D productivity: the pharmaceutical industry's grand challenge. *Nat Rev Drug Discov.* 2010;9(3):203–214.
3. Scott CW, Peters MF, Dragan YP. Human induced pluripotent stem cells and their use in drug discovery for toxicity testing. *Toxicol Lett.* 2013;219(1):49–58.
4. Van Norman GA. Limitations of animal studies for predicting toxicity in clinical trials: is it time to rethink our current approach? *JACC Basic Transl Sci.* 2019;4(7):845–854.
5. Day CP, Merlino G, Van Dyke T. Preclinical mouse cancer models: a maze of opportunities and challenges. *Cell.* 2015;163(1):39–53.
6. Tian C, Qin T, Liu W, Wang J. Recent advances in microfluidic technologies for organ-on-a-chip. *TrAC Trends Anal Chem.* 2019;117:146–156. doi:10.1016/j.trac.2019.06.005.
7. Bhatia S, Ingber D. Microfluidic organs-on-chips. *Nat Biotechnol.* 2014;32:760–772. doi:10.1038/nbt.2989.
8. Ramadan Q, Zourob M. Organ-on-a-chip engineering: toward bridging the gap between lab and industry. *Biomicrofluidics.* 2020 Jul 14;14(4):041501. doi:10.1063/5.0011583. PMID: 32699563; PMCID: PMC7367691.
9. Zhang B, Korolj A, Lai BF, Radisic M. Advances in organ-on-a-chip engineering. *Nat Rev Mater.* 2018;3(8):257–278.
10. Cheriyedath S. What Is Microfluidics? News-Medical.net. 2024. https://www.news-medical.net/life-sciences/What-is-Microfluidics.aspx. Accessed 2024 Jan 14.
11. Huh D, Matthews BD, Mammoto A, Montoya-Zavala M, Hsin HY, Ingber DE. Reconstituting organ-level lung functions on a chip. *Science.* 2010 Jun 25;328(5986):1662–1668. doi:10.1126/science.1188302. PMID: 20576885; PMCID: PMC8335790.
12. Mathur A, Loskill P, Shao K, Huebsch N, Hong SG, Marcus SG, et al. Human iPSC-based cardiac microphysiological system for drug screening applications. *Sci Rep.* 2015;9:5:8883. doi:10.1038/srep08883.

13. Bovard D, Sandoz A, Luettich K, Frentzel S, Iskandar A, Marescotti D, et al. A lung/liver-on-a-chip platform for acute and chronic toxicity studies. *Lab Chip*. 2018;18(24):3814–3829. doi:10.1039/C8LC01029C.

14. Kim HJ, Li H, Collins JJ, Ingber DE. Contributions of microbiome and mechanical deformation to intestinal bacterial overgrowth and inflammation in a human gut-on-a-chip. *Proc Natl Acad Sci U S A*. 2016 Jan 5;113(1): E7–15. doi:10.1073/pnas.1522193112. Epub 2015 Dec 14. PMID: 26668389; PMCID: PMC4711860.

15. Lee-Montiel FT, Laemmle A, Charwat V, Dumon L, Lee CS, Huebsch N, et al. Integrated isogenic human induced pluripotent stem cell-based liver and heart microphysiological systems predict unsafe drug-drug interaction. *Front Pharmacol*. 2021 May 7;12:667010. doi:10.3389/fphar.2021.667010. PMID: 34025426; PMCID: PMC8138446.

16. Mariano A, Conficconi C, Lemme M, Occhetta P, Gaudiello E, Votta E, et al. Beating heart on a chip: a novel microfluidic platform to generate functional 3D cardiac microtissues. *Lab Chip*. 2016;16(3):599–610. doi:10.1039/c5lc01356a.

17. Zhu J. Application of organ-on-chip in drug discovery. *J Biosci Med*. 2020;08(03). doi:10.4236/jbm.2020.83011.

18. Low LA, Tagle DA. Tissue chips — innovative tools for drug development and disease modeling. *Lab Chip*. 2017 Sep 12;17(18):3026–3036. doi:10.1039/c7lc00462a. PMID: 28795174; PMCID: PMC5621042.

19. Huh DD. A human breathing lung-on-a-chip. *Ann Am Thorac Soc*. 2015 Mar;12(Suppl 1):S42–S44. doi:10.1513/AnnalsATS.201410-442MG. PMID: 25830834; PMCID: PMC5467107.

20. Skardal A, Murphy SV, Devarasetty M, Mead I, Kang W, Seol YJ, et al. Multi-tissue interactions in an integrated three-tissue organ-on-a-chip platform. *Sci Rep*. 2017;7(1):8837. doi:10.1038/s41598-017-08879-x.

21. Deng S, Li C, Cao J, Cui Z, Du J, Fu Z, Yang H, Chen P. Organ-on-a-chip meets artificial intelligence in drug evaluation. *Theranostics*. 2023 Aug 15;13(13):4526–4558. doi:10.7150/thno.87266. PMID: 37649608; PMCID: PMC10465229.

22. van der Meer AD, van den Berg A. Organs-on-chips: breaking the in vitro impasse. *Integr Biol (Camb)*. 2012;4(5):461–470. doi:10.1039/c2ib00176d.

23. Esch EW, Bahinski A, Huh D. Organs-on-chips at the frontiers of drug discovery. *Nat Rev Drug Discov*. 2015 Apr;14(4):248–260. doi:10.1038/nrd4539. Epub 2015 Mar 20. PMID: 25792263; PMCID: PMC4826389.

24. Imparato G, Urciuolo F, Netti PA. Organ on chip technology to model cancer growth and metastasis. *Bioengineering (Basel).* 2022 Jan 11; 9(1):28. doi:10.3390/bioengineering9010028. PMID: 35049737; PMCID: PMC8772984.
25. Akhtar A, Andleeb A, Sher Waris T, Bazzar M, Moradi AR, Awan NR, et al., Neurodegenerative diseases and effective drug delivery: a review of challenges and novel therapeutics. *J Control Release.* 2020;330:1152–1167. doi:10.1016/j.jconrel.2020.11.021.
26. Milne CP. *CNS Drugs Take 20% Longer to Develop and to Approve vs. Non-CNS Drugs.* Boston: Tufts Center for the Study of Drug Development. 2018. https://www.globenewswire.com/news-release/2018/09/11/1569156/0/en/CNS-Drugs-Take-20-Longer-to-Develop-and-38-Longer-to-Approve-vs-Non-CNS-Drugs-According-to-the-Tufts-Center-for-the-Study-of-Drug-Development.html.
27. Spitz S, Ko E, Ertl P, Kamm RD. How organ-on-a-chip technology can assist in studying the role of the glymphatic system in neurodegenerative diseases. *Int J Mol Sci.* 2023;24(3):2171. doi:10.3390/ijms24032171.
28. Ma C, Peng Y, Li H, Chen W. Organ-on-a-chip: a new paradigm for drug development. *Trends Pharmacol Sci.* 2021 Feb;42(2):119–133. doi:10.1016/j.tips.2020.11.009. Epub 2020 Dec 16. PMID: 33341248; PMCID: PMC7990030.
29. Ashammakhi N, Elmusrati M. An array of gut-on-a-chips for drug development. *BioRxiv.* 2018;273847.
30. Perelson AS, Ribeiro RM. Introduction to modeling viral infections and immunity. *Immunol Rev.* 2018;285(1):5–8.
31. Hartung T. Toxicity testing in the 21st century. *Nature.* 2009;460:208–212.
32. Shahabipour F, Satta S, Mahmoodi M, Sun A, de Barros NR, Li S, et al. Engineering organ-on-a-chip systems to model viral infections. *Biofabrication.* 2023 Feb 6;15(2). doi:10.1088/1758-5090/ac6538. PMID: 35390777; PMCID: PMC9883621.
33. Xian C, Zhang J, Zhao S, Li XG. Gut-on-a-chip for disease models. *J Tissue Eng.* 2023 Jan 18;14. doi:10.1177/20417314221149882. PMID: 36699635; PMCID: PMC9869227.
34. Beaurivage C, Kanapeckaite A, Loomans C, Erdmann KS, Stallen J, Janssen RAJ. Development of a human primary gut-on-a-chip to model inflammatory processes. *Sci Rep.* 2020;10(1):21475. doi:10.1038/s41598-020-78359-2.

35. Thacker VV, Sharma K, Dhar N, Mancini GF, Sordet-Dessimoz J, McKinney JD. Rapid endotheliitis and vascular damage characterize SARS-CoV-2 infection in a human lung-on-chip model. *EMBO Rep.* 2021;22(6):e52744.

36. Maulana TI, Kromidas E, Wallstabe L, Cipriano M, Alb M, Zaupa C, et al. Immunocompetent cancer-on-chip models to assess immuno-oncology therapy. *Adv Drug Deliv Rev.* 2021;173:281–305. doi:10.1016/j.addr.2021.03.015. https://www.sciencedirect.com/science/article/pii/S0169409X21000934.

37. Tibbitt MW, Anseth KS. Hydrogels as extracellular matrix mimics for 3D cell culture. *Biotechnol Bioeng.* 2009 Jul 1;103(4):655–663. doi:10.1002/bit.22361. PMID: 19472329; PMCID: PMC2997742.

38. Mastrangeli M, Millet S, ORCHID partners T, van den Eijnden-van Raaij J. Organ-on-chip in development: towards a roadmap for organs-on-chip. *ALTEX.* 2019;36(4):650–668. doi:10.14573/altex.1908271.

39. Ribas J, Sadeghi H, Manbachi A, Leijten J, Brinegar K, Zhang YS, et al. Cardiovascular organ-on-a-chip platforms for drug discovery and development. *Appl Vitro Toxicol.* 2016 Jun 1;2(2):82–96. doi:10.1089/aivt.2016.0002. PMID: 28971113; PMCID: PMC5044977.

40. Annabi N, Selimović Š, Acevedo Cox JP, Ribas J, Bakooshli A, Heintze D, et al. Hydrogel-coated microfluidic channels for cardiomyocyte culture. *Lab Chip.* 2013;13:3569–3577.

41. Duffy DC, McDonald JC, Schueller OJ, Whitesides GM. Rapid prototyping of microfluidic systems in poly(dimethylsiloxane). *Anal Chem.* 1998;70(23):4974–4984.

42. Halldorsson S, Lucumi E, Gómez-Sjöberg R, Fleming RMT. Advantages and challenges of microfluidic cell culture in polydimethylsiloxane devices. *Biosens Bioelectron.* 2015;63:218–231.

43. Shi Y, Inoue H, Wu JC, Yamanaka S. Induced pluripotent stem cell technology: a decade of progress. *Nat. Rev. Drug Discov.* 2017;16(2):115–130.

44. van den Berg A, Mummery CL, Passier R, van der Meer AD. Personalised organs-on-chips: functional testing for precision medicine. *Lab Chip.* 2019;19(2):198–205.

45. Zakrzewski W, Dobrzyński M, Szymonowicz M, Rybak Z. Stem cells: Past, present, and future. *Stem Cell Res Ther.* 2019 Feb 26;10(1):68. doi:10.1186/s13287-019-1165-5. PMID: 30808416; PMCID: PMC6390367.

46. Sung JH, Esch MB, Prot JM, et al. Microfabricated mammalian organ systems and their integration into models of whole animals and humans. *Lab Chip.* 2013;13(7):1201–1212. doi:10.1039/c3lc41017j.

47. Maschmeyer I, Lorenz AK, Schimek K, Hasenberg T, Ramme AP, Hübner J, et al. A four-organ-chip for interconnected long-term co-culture of human intestine, liver, skin and kidney equivalents. *Lab Chip*. 2015;15(12):2688–2699. doi:10.1039/C5LC00392J.

48. Wagner I, Materne EM, Brincker S, Süssbier U, Frädrich C, Busek M, et al. A dynamic multi-organ-chip for long-term cultivation and substance testing proven by 3D human liver and skin tissue co-culture. *Lab Chip*. 2013;13(18):3538–3547. doi:10.1039/c3lc50234a.

49. Mastrangeli M, Millet S, Mummery C, Loskill P, Braeken D, Eberle W, et al. Building blocks for a European organ-on-chip roadmap. *ALTEX*. 2019;36(3):481–492. doi:10.14573/altex.1905221.

50. Marx U, Akabane T, Andersson TB, Baker E, Beilmann M, Beken S, et al. Biology-inspired microphysiological systems to advance patient benefit and animal welfare in drug development. *ALTEX*. 2020;37(3):365–394. doi:10.14573/altex.2001241. Epub 2020 Feb 28. PMID: 32113184; PMCID: PMC7863570

51. Schneider MR, Oelgeschlaeger M, Burgdorf T, van Meer P, Theunissen P, Kienhuis AS, et al. Applicability of organ-on-chip systems in toxicology and pharmacology. *Crit Rev Toxico*. 2021;51(6):540–554. doi:10.1080/10408444.2021.1953439.

52. Teixeira SG, Houeto P, Gattacceca F, Petitcollot N, Debruyne D, Guerbet M, et al. National reflection on organs-on-chip for drug development: new regulatory challenges. *Toxicol Lett*. 2032;388:1–12. doi:10.1016/j.toxlet.2023.09.011. https://www.sciencedirect.com/science/article/pii/S0378427423010548.

53. Unlock Human-Relevant Insights with Organ-Chips. Emulate. https://emulatebio.com/?utm_source=google&utm_medium=cpc&utm_campaign=Unbranded_General&utm_term=organ_on_a_chip&utm_term=organ%20on%20a%20chip&utm_source=adwords&utm_medium=ppc&utm_campaign=Unbranded+General&hsa_cam=18716528387&hsa_grp=144253413793&hsa_mt=e&hsa_src=g&hsa_ad=630861078857&hsa_acc=8851317517&hsa_net=adwords&hsa_kw=organ%20on%20a%20chip&hsa_tgt=kwd-329009267684&hsa_ver=3&gad_source=1&gclid=CjwKCAiAzJOtBhALEiwAtwj8trmiSm_ns1JTrwS6TWhpXI-oCrv0N0700k5vyqNoAr3prwPXGPlSdFhoCNKwQAvD_BwE. Accessed 2024 Jan 15.

Chapter 7

3D Organ Printing: Transforming Transplantation and Tissue Repair

Introduction

Brief Overview of 3D Organ Printing

Three-dimensional (3D) organ printing, a remarkable fusion of biology, technology, and medicine, stands at the forefront of one of the most exciting advancements in healthcare. This innovative process involves creating 3D, functional biological structures — such as tissues and organs — layer by layer from bioinks, biomaterials containing living cells. The technology leverages principles from traditional 3D printing, adapted to handle the complexities of human biology.

At its core, 3D organ printing utilizes specialized printers that deposit layers of cells and biocompatible materials in precise configurations. These layers, guided by digital models, gradually build up to form structures that closely mimic the natural composition of human tissues and organs. The process involves a meticulous orchestration of cell types, growth factors, and scaffolding materials to ensure the viability and functionality of the printed organs.

The Significance of this Technology in Modern Medicine

The implications of 3D organ printing in modern medicine are profound. This technology addresses one of the most pressing challenges in healthcare:

the shortage of organ donors for transplantation. 3D organ printing could drastically reduce transplant waiting lists and the associated complications of immune rejection by providing a source of personalized organs.

Moreover, the applications for 3D organ printing transcend transplantation. It opens new avenues in pharmaceutical research and drug testing, allowing for more accurate and ethical testing methods by reducing reliance on animal models. Researchers can use printed tissues to study disease mechanisms, test drug efficacy, and explore new treatments in a controlled and patient-specific manner.

In tissue repair and regenerative medicine, 3D organ printing offers solutions for reconstructive surgeries, particularly in cases of severe injuries or congenital defects. The ability to print tissues that precisely match a patient's anatomy and cellular composition can lead to more effective and personalized treatments.

3D organ printing is a technological marvel and a beacon of hope in medicine. It promises to revolutionize transplantation, drug development, and tissue repair, creating a new era where personalized and accessible healthcare solutions are a reality.

Understanding 3D Printing Technology

Basic Principles of 3D Printing

3D printing, or additive manufacturing, creates 3D objects from a digital file. It involves adding a material layer by layer to build a final product. This contrasts with traditional subtractive manufacturing methods, where the material is removed from a solid block to achieve the desired shape. The basic steps in 3D printing include designing a 3D model in a computer-aided design (CAD) program, slicing the model into thin horizontal layers, and then sequentially printing these layers to form the complete object.

Evolution from Manufacturing to Bioprinting

Initially developed for industrial applications, 3D printing has evolved to encompass bioprinting, a specialized form of 3D printing that uses living cells and biomaterials to create tissue-like structures. This evolution was driven by

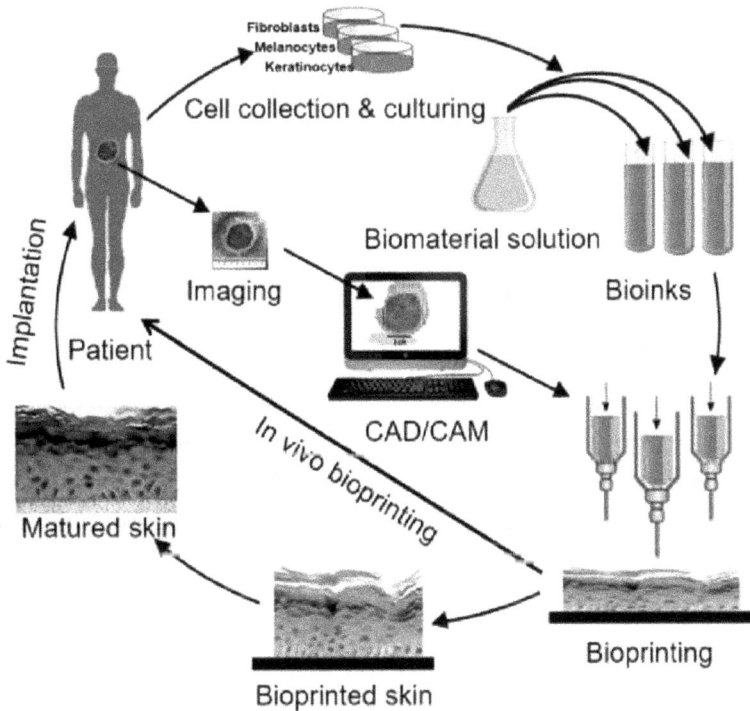

Figure 1. Bioprinting process for skin repair.

the need for more complex and biologically relevant models in medical research and the demand for personalized medical solutions. Bioprinting leverages the foundational principles of 3D printing but introduces biological components, making it a more complex and delicate process. See Figure 1.

For example, researchers at the Wake Forest Institute for Regenerative Medicine have pioneered bioprinting, demonstrating the potential to print skin cells onto burn wounds.[1]

Fundamental Components: Bioinks, Printers, and Scaffolds

The orchestration of bioinks, printers, and scaffolds forms the cornerstone of 3D bioprinting, a transformative technology.

Bioinks

Bioinks play a pivotal role in 3D bioprinting, serving as the fundamental medium through which living tissues are fabricated. These specialized inks blend biological components that must meet several critical criteria to effectively create viable, functional tissues.

Composition of Bioinks

Cellular Component

The primary component of bioinks is living cells. See Figure 2. These can be various cell types, including stem cells, which have the potential to differentiate into specific tissue cells or mature cells derived from the tissue of interest. The choice of cells depends on the target tissue or organ.

Polymeric Matrix

Cells in bioinks are suspended in a hydrogel matrix typically composed of natural or synthetic polymers. Natural polymers, such as alginate, collagen,

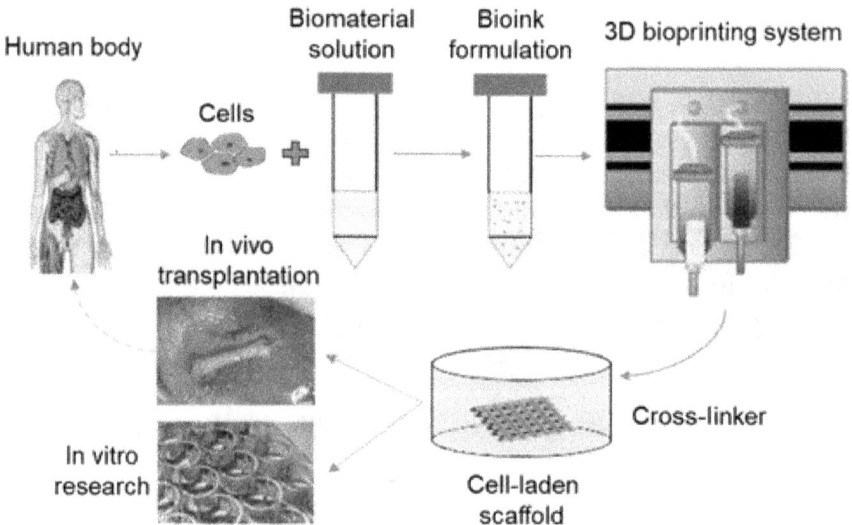

Figure 2.   Bioink development and utilization.

gelatin, and fibrin, are often preferred due to their biocompatibility and ability to mimic the natural extracellular matrix (ECM). Synthetic polymers, such as polyethylene glycol (PEG), can be engineered to have specific properties but may lack the bioactivity of natural materials.

A study by Gao et al.[2] demonstrated the successful use of a gelatin methacryloyl (GelMA) hydrogel in bioinks, highlighting its suitability for cell encapsulation and tissue engineering due to its tunable mechanical properties and biocompatibility.[3]

Requirements for Effective Bioinks

Biocompatibility

The bioink must be nontoxic and support cell viability, proliferation, and differentiation. It should also allow for exchanging nutrients and waste to keep the cells healthy.

Mechanical Properties

The bioink should possess mechanical properties conducive to the printing process and the stability of the printed structure. It needs the appropriate viscosity to facilitate extrusion, maintain its shape, and support the cells until they can produce their own ECM and stabilize the tissue. The bioink should also have the mechanical strength to provide structural support and the flexibility to allow deformation without breaking.

Printability

Good printability is essential for bioinks to ensure precise deposition of the material and high-resolution tissue structures. This includes appropriate viscosity and gelation properties that allow the ink to flow through the printer nozzle and solidify in the desired pattern.

Degradation Rate

The bioink degradation rate should match the tissue maturation rate. As the printed tissue develops, the scaffold material should degrade at a rate that allows for the gradual transfer of mechanical load to the developing tissue.

Challenges and Innovations

Developing the ideal bioink is a complex task, and researchers continually experiment with different formulations to enhance their performance. Innovations in bioink design include incorporating growth factors, developing composite materials combining the best properties of natural and synthetic polymers, and using advanced techniques such as decellularized ECM components to provide a more native tissue-like environment. See Figure 3.

For example, a study by Skylar-Scott et al.[4] demonstrated using a novel bioink formulation for creating vascularized cardiac tissues.

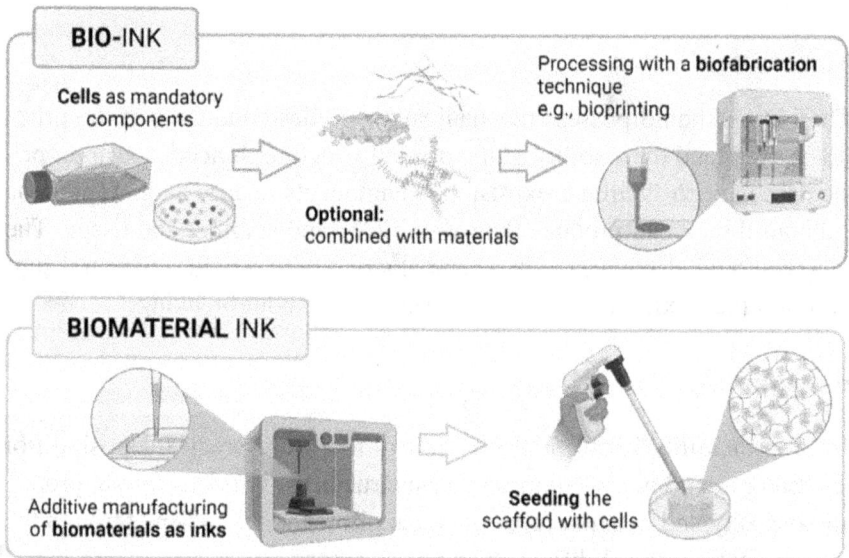

BIO-INK

Cells as mandatory components

Processing with a **biofabrication** technique e.g., bioprinting

Optional: combined with materials

BIOMATERIAL INK

Additive manufacturing of **biomaterials as inks**

Seeding the scaffold with cells

Figure 3. Two techniques for bioprinting: incorporating cells into a hydrogel for extrusion in a bioprinter (top) and creating a scaffold in a bioprinter first and then seeding the scaffold with cells (bottom).

Bioprinters

Bioprinters are specialized devices at the heart of 3D organ printing technology. They are crucial in the precise and controlled bioink deposition to create complex tissue structures. The functionality and sophistication of bioprinters are central to the success of 3D bioprinting processes. See Figure 4.

The Integrated Tissue and Organ Printing System (ITOP), developed at the Wake Forest, is an example of a high-precision bioprinter capable of printing human-scale tissues.[5]

Types of Bioprinters

Inkjet-Based Bioprinters

These printers function similarly to traditional inkjet printers but use bioinks instead of conventional ink. Inkjet-based printers use thermal or acoustic energy to deposit bioink droplets onto a substrate layer by layer. Inkjet bioprinters are known for their high speed and ability to print with relatively high resolution. However, they may be less suitable for highly viscous bioinks or applications requiring the deposition of large cell volumes.

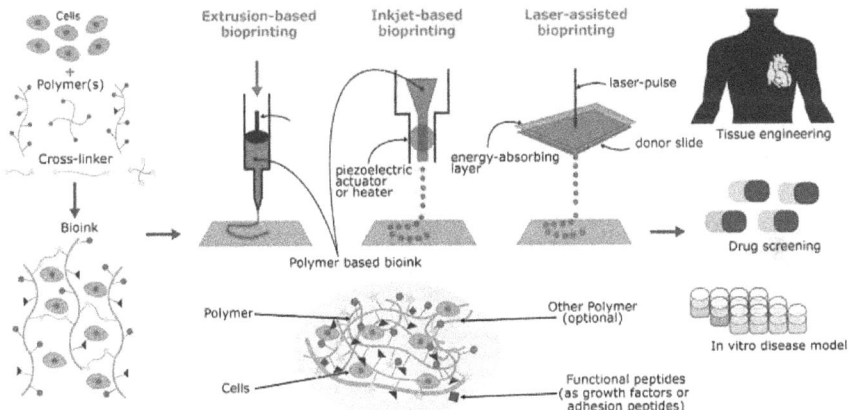

Figure 4. 3D bioprinting process.

Inkjet bioprinting has created layered skin tissue constructs using Chinese hamster ovary cells and embryonic motor neuron cells in predefined patterns.[4]

Another example of inkjet-based bioprinting is the work by Organovo, which specializes in developing functional human tissues using 3D bioprinting technology. They have successfully printed liver tissues that are used for drug toxicity testing, providing a more accurate and ethical alternative to animal testing.[6]

Extrusion-Based Bioprinters

These printers use a continuous flow of bioink extruded through one or more nozzles. This type is more versatile regarding the range of bioinks it can handle, including highly viscous materials. Extrusion bioprinters can create more structurally robust tissues but often at a lower resolution than inkjet printers. However, the pressure and shear stress during extrusion can be challenging for cell viability. See Figure 5.

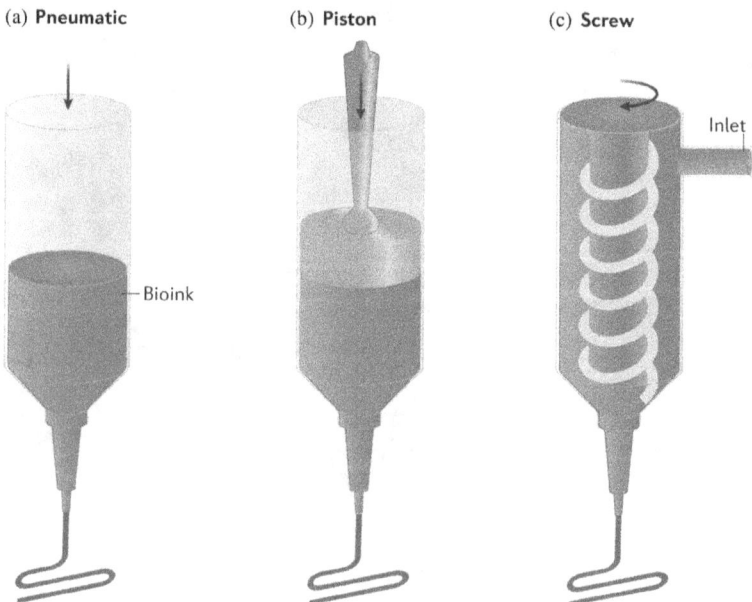

Figure 5. Three types of extrusion printers.

A notable example of extrusion-based bioprinting is the work done by researchers at the University of Toronto. They developed a skin bioprinter that precisely places skin cells onto wounds to improve healing. This bioprinter deposited layers of skin tissue directly onto a wound, significantly aiding the healing process.[7]

An extrusion-based bioprinter was also used to fabricate a functional human-scale bone and cartilage structure.[8]

Laser-Assisted Bioprinters

In this type of printer, a laser pulse is used to deposit bioink onto the substrate. This method is known for its high precision and minimal mechanical stress on the cells, making it suitable for sensitive cell types. However, laser-assisted bioprinters can be more complex and costly.

An example of laser-assisted bioprinting can be seen in the work conducted by Poietis, a French biotechnology company. They have developed a laser-assisted bioprinting technology to create complex tissue models, including multilayered skin and bone tissues.[9]

Vital Functional Requirements of Bioprinters

1. Precision and Accuracy: Bioprinters must deposit cells and biomaterials with high precision to replicate the complex architecture of natural tissues. This includes accurate control over the size and placement of each printed droplet or filament.
2. Cell Viability: The printing process must maintain high cell viability. This involves gentle handling of the bioink to avoid damaging the cells during printing. Parameters such as temperature, pressure, and shear forces must be carefully controlled.
3. Speed and Efficiency: Precision and cell viability are paramount, but printing must also be efficient. A balance must be struck between the printing speed and the printed tissues' resolution and viability.
4. Compatibility with Bioinks: Bioprinters must be compatible with various bioinks, each having different properties and requirements. This includes handling varying viscosities and compositions without clogging or damaging the bioink.

Challenges and Innovations

Developing bioprinters that meet all these requirements is a significant engineering challenge. Innovations in this field include the development of multinozzle systems that can print different types of cells and materials simultaneously and the integration of real-time monitoring systems to adjust printing parameters for optimal cell viability and tissue formation.

Bioprinters are sophisticated devices that require a high degree of precision and control to successfully create viable, functional tissues. The ongoing advancements in bioprinter technology are crucial for the continued growth and success of 3D organ printing in regenerative medicine and tissue engineering.

Scaffolds

Scaffolds in bioprinting play a critical role in the successful creation of functional tissues and organs. They serve as a temporary framework that supports the cells during the initial stages of tissue formation and maturation. The design and composition of these scaffolds are crucial, as they must meet several key requirements to ensure the viability and proper functioning of the printed tissues.

Composition and Properties of Scaffolds

1. Biocompatibility: Scaffolds must be made from biocompatible materials, meaning they do not provoke an immune response or cause toxicity in the body. This ensures that the scaffold can integrate seamlessly with the body's tissues without causing inflammation or rejection.
2. Biodegradability: An essential feature of scaffolds in bioprinting is their biodegradability. They are designed to degrade at a rate that matches the growth and development of the new tissue. As the cells proliferate and start forming their ECM, the scaffold gradually dissolves, leaving behind a fully functional tissue or organ. The degradation products should be nontoxic and safely absorbed or excreted by the body.

3. Mechanical Strength and Flexibility: The scaffold must possess adequate mechanical strength to maintain structural integrity during the printing process and initial tissue formation. It should also have enough flexibility to mimic the mechanical properties of the natural tissue it is replacing or supporting.

4. Pore Structure and Size: The porosity of the scaffold, including the pore size and distribution, is critical for cell migration, nutrient and oxygen diffusion, and waste removal. A well-designed pore structure facilitates vascularization, which is essential for the survival of thicker tissues.

Materials used in Scaffold Design

1. Natural Polymers: Materials such as collagen, gelatin, alginate, fibrin, and chitosan are commonly used due to their excellent biocompatibility and biodegradability. They closely mimic the natural ECM, promoting cell attachment and growth.

2. Synthetic Polymers: Polymers such as polylactic acid (PLA), polyglycolic acid (PGA), and polycaprolactone (PCL) are used for their tunable degradation rates and mechanical properties. They can be engineered to meet specific requirements of different tissues.

3. Composite Materials: Combining natural and synthetic polymers can create scaffolds that possess both the biocompatibility of natural materials and the mechanical stability of synthetic ones. This approach allows for the customization of scaffolds for specific applications.

Challenges and Innovations

Developing scaffolds that meet all these requirements is a significant challenge. Innovations in scaffold design include incorporating growth factors or other bioactive molecules to promote tissue growth and using advanced fabrication techniques to create more complex and precise structures. See Figure 6.

A study by Murphy and Atala[6] discusses various materials used for scaffolds in bioprinting. These include gel-cast hydroxyapatite (HA)

Step 1. Bioprinting of microfibrous scaffold encapsulating endothelial cells.   **Step 2.** Formation of the endothelialized structure and the vascular bed.

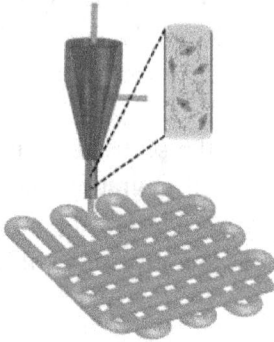

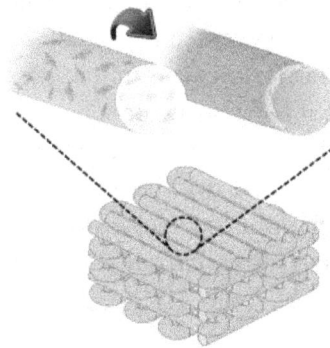

Step 3. Seeding with cardiomyocytes.   **Step 4.** Formation of endothelialized myocardium.

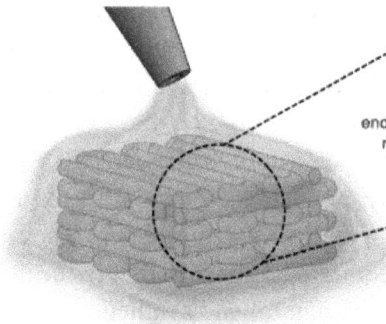

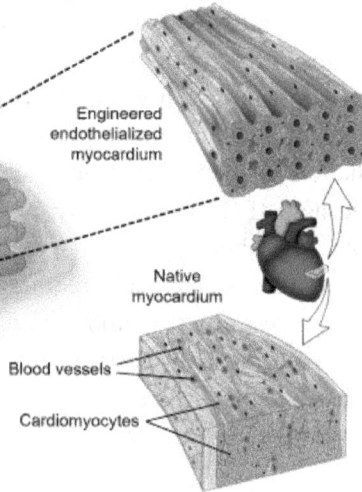

Engineered
endothelialized
myocardium

Native
myocardium

Blood vessels

Cardiomyocytes

Figure 6.   Creating a scaffold of donor cells to mimic human myocardial tissues.

foams, bioactive glass foam, and biodegradable polymer foam, as well as the "electrospinning" of polymers to form an electrostatic field that mimics the structure and physiochemical features of natural fibers. These materials and techniques highlight the importance of scaffold design in tissue engineering.[6] See Figure 7.

In another example, a study by Hospodiuk et al.[10] highlighted the use of a composite scaffold made from a blend of gelatin and PCL,

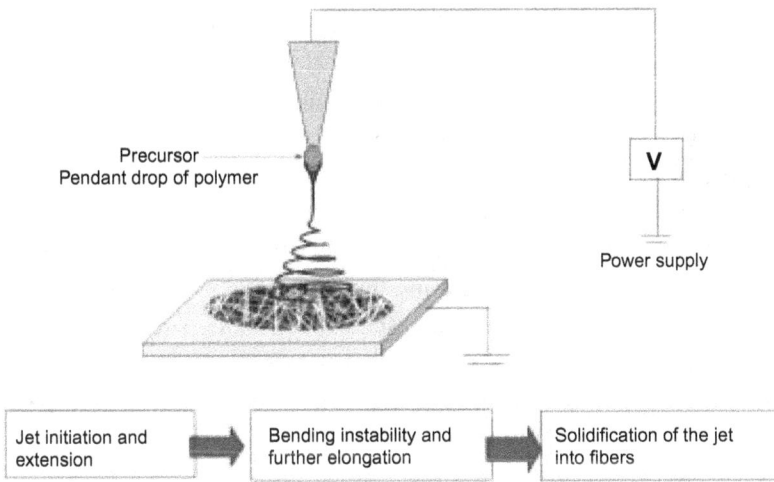

Figure 7. Electrospinning fibers for bioprinted scaffolding.

demonstrating improved cell viability and structural integrity for tissue engineering applications.

Scaffolds in bioprinting are fundamental to the creation of viable, functional tissues and organs. Their design and material composition are critical to supporting cell growth, tissue development, and integration with the body, making them a key area of focus in the field of 3D bioprinting.

3D organ printing, as we can see, is evolving from traditional manufacturing to bioprinting, and it involves complex interplays between bioinks, printers, and scaffolds. Each component plays a crucial role in creating viable, functional tissues and organs, marking a significant advancement in medical technology and treatment possibilities.

The Science behind 3D Organ Printing

Cell Biology in Organ Printing: Stem Cells and Differentiated Cells

The foundation of 3D organ printing lies in cell biology, specifically the use of stem cells and differentiated cells.

1. Stem Cells: These are undifferentiated cells capable of transforming into various cell types, making them ideal for organ printing. Stem cells can be sourced from embryos (embryonic stem cells) or adult tissues (adult stem cells). Induced pluripotent stem cells (iPSCs), derived by reprogramming adult cells to an embryonic-like state, are particularly valuable due to their versatility and patient-specific nature.

   iPSCs have been used to create complex structures such as vascularized heart tissues, demonstrating their potential in organ printing.[11]

2. Differentiated Cells: These are specialized cells, such as cardiac or liver cells, used to print tissues that require specific functions. The source of these cells can be primary tissues or stem cells that have been differentiated into the desired cell type.

Process of Creating Bioinks

Bioinks, which contain living cells, are the materials used in 3D bioprinting. The process of creating bioinks involves the following steps:

1. Cell Selection and Preparation: Choosing the right type of cells based on the tissue or organ to be printed. Cells are then cultured and expanded to obtain a sufficient quantity for the proposed application.

2. Hydrogel Formation: Cells are mixed with a hydrogel matrix, which provides structural support. Hydrogels are chosen based on their biocompatibility, mechanical properties, and degradation rates. Common hydrogels include collagen, alginate, and fibrin.

3. Optimization for Printing: The bioink must have the right viscosity and flow properties for printing. This often involves fine-tuning the concentration of cells and hydrogel components.

Applications in Medicine

3D organ printing, a groundbreaking technology in the field of regenerative medicine, has opened new possibilities in various medical applications. This section explores its significant contributions to tissue repair and regeneration, organ transplantation, and personalized medicine.

Tissue Repair and Regeneration: Skin, Bone, and Cartilage

Skin

3D bioprinting in skin regeneration represents a significant advancement in medical technology, particularly for the treatment of burns, chronic wounds, and skin diseases. This technology involves the layer-by-layer precise deposition of biological materials, such as cells and growth factors, to create tissue-like structures that mimic natural skin. A study by Cubo et al.[12] demonstrated the successful application of a 3D bioprinter to create human skin, showing potential for immediate clinical use in burn treatment and wound healing.

Here are the key aspects of this technology:

Customization

One of the primary benefits of 3D bioprinted skin grafts is their ability to be customized to the patient's specific needs. This includes matching the size, depth, and structure of the wound, which is crucial for effective healing. Traditional skin grafts, in contrast, are limited by the availability and suitability of donor skin.

Cellular Composition

Bioprinted skin can be composed of different types of cells, such as keratinocytes, fibroblasts, and even melanocytes, to closely replicate the natural skin layers. This can lead to better integration and functionality of the graft.

Growth Factors and Bioinks

The use of specialized bioinks, which are biomaterials that support cell growth and differentiation, is crucial. These bioinks can be enriched with growth factors that promote wound healing and tissue regeneration.

Reduced Rejection Risk

Since bioprinted skin can be created using the patient's cells, the risk of immune rejection is significantly reduced compared to traditional skin grafts from donors.

Applications in Chronic Wounds and Burns

For patients with chronic wounds, such as diabetic ulcers, or extensive burns, bioprinted skin offers a promising treatment option. It can provide a faster and more effective healing process compared to conventional treatments.

Research and Development

While the technology is promising, it is still largely in the research and development phase. Clinical trials are necessary to fully understand the efficacy and safety of bioprinted skin grafts.

Ethical and Regulatory Considerations

The development and application of bioprinted skin also involve ethical and regulatory considerations, including approval from medical regulatory bodies and addressing any ethical concerns related to the use of human cells.

Cost and Accessibility

Currently, the cost of 3D bioprinting technology is high, which may limit its accessibility. However, as the technology advances and becomes more widespread, costs are expected to decrease.

3D bioprinting for skin regeneration holds great promise for improving the treatment of burns, chronic wounds, and skin diseases. It offers customization, reduced rejection risk, and the potential for enhanced healing. However, it is important to continue research and address ethical, regulatory, and cost issues to fully realize its potential.

Bone

Bioprinting for bone repair is an emerging area in regenerative medicine that addresses the challenges associated with complex or nonhealing fractures. This technology utilizes 3D printing techniques to create bone scaffolds that are infused with bioinks containing osteogenic cells and growth factors.

Bioinks used in bone bioprinting are specialized materials that can support the growth and differentiation of osteogenic cells, such as osteoblasts. These cells are essential for bone formation and healing.

The inclusion of growth factors in bioinks is crucial. These substances, such as bone morphogenetic proteins (BMPs), stimulate bone growth and help in the integration of the bioprinted scaffold with the patient's existing bone tissue.[13]

The scaffolds created through bioprinting are designed to mimic the complex structure of natural bone. They provide a temporary matrix for bone growth and are engineered to degrade safely as new bone tissue forms.[14]

Bioprinting allows for the customization of the scaffold to match the specific size, shape, and mechanical properties required for individual patients and fracture types. This is particularly beneficial for complex fractures where traditional treatments may be inadequate. A study by Kang et al.[5] in the journal *Nature Biotechnology* demonstrated the use of a 3D-printed hyperelastic "bone" that could be easily customized for bone implants.

Research by Kang et al.[5] involved 3D printing of a bone scaffold embedded with human mesenchymal stem cells, demonstrating the potential for bone regeneration.

One of the challenges in bone bioprinting is ensuring the mechanical strength and stability of the printed scaffold to withstand the stresses in the bone repair site. Lee et al. addressed this problem by developing a composite bioink for 3D printing of a scaffold for bone tissue engineering. These researchers were able to control the morphology of the scaffolds. This new morphology was able to control the alignment, proliferation, and adhesion of osteoblasts. This improved the quality and quantity of the regenerated bone.[15]

Bioceramics such as HA and tricalcium phosphate are used in bone tissue engineering, for their osteoconductivity and similarity to bone mineral.[16]

Osteoconductivity can be described as the property of a material to support tissue ingrowth, osteoprogenitor cell growth, and development for bone formation to occur. The appropriate architectural geometry and chemical composition are the important features of osteoconductivity.[17,18]

Future research will focus on improving the vascularization within the bioprinted structures to ensure the survival and integration of the printed bone tissue.

Bioprinting offers a promising approach to bone repair, especially for complex and nonhealing fractures. The ability to customize scaffolds with bioinks infused with osteogenic cells and growth factors could revolutionize the treatment of bone injuries.

Cartilage

3D bioprinting for cartilage repair, especially in joints, is a burgeoning area in regenerative medicine. The technology's ability to create cartilage scaffolds that replicate the intricate structure and mechanical properties of native cartilage offers significant potential for treating joint disorders, such as osteoarthritis or cartilage damage from injuries.

Cartilage is a resilient and smooth elastic tissue, a rubber-like padding that covers and protects the ends of long bones at the joints. Its complex structure is difficult to replicate with traditional methods, making bioprinting a particularly promising approach.

3D bioprinting can produce scaffolds that mimic the unique mechanical and structural properties of cartilage. These scaffolds can be infused with cells, such as chondrocytes (the cells found in healthy cartilage), and growth factors that promote cartilage regeneration.[19] See Figure 8.

Bioprinting allows for the customization of the scaffold to fit the specific shape and size of the damaged cartilage area in a patient's joint, which is crucial for successful repair and functionality. A study by Daly et al.[20] in the *Biofabrication* journal demonstrated the potential of 3D bioprinting for creating complex, zonally organized cartilage tissue constructs.[21]

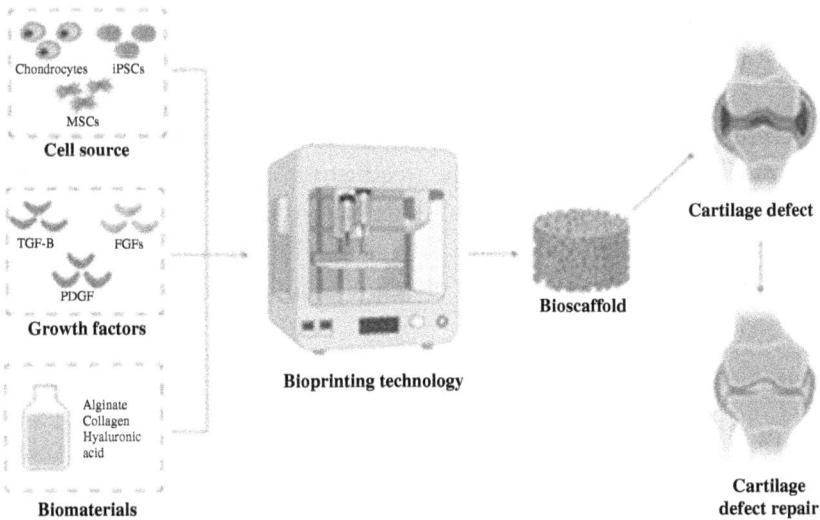

Figure 8. Using a bioprinted scaffold to create cartilage for joint repair.

Specifically, they used inkjet bioprinting to deposit defined numbers of mesenchymal stromal cells (MSCs) and chondrocytes into preprinted microchambers. The composition and biomechanical properties of the resulting bioprinted cartilage were comparable to native tissue. Mouser et al.[22] in the *Journal of Biomedical Materials Research* explored the use of 3D bioprinting for fabricating anatomically shaped cartilage constructs using MRI data, showcasing the potential for patient-specific treatments.

One of the main challenges in bioprinting cartilage is replicating the tissue's mechanical properties, such as its ability to withstand compressive and tensile forces.[23]

A study by Daly et al.[20] highlighted the use of 3D bioprinting to create scaffolds for knee cartilage repair, using a combination of cells and bio-materials to mimic the mechanical properties of cartilage.

Ensuring the long-term viability and integration of the bioprinted cartilage within the joint environment is also a critical area of focus. If successful, bioprinted cartilage could provide a solution for patients suffering from joint pain, immobility, or cartilage degradation, reducing the need for more invasive procedures such as joint replacements. As with other bioprinting applications, cartilage repair strategies must navigate regulatory pathways to ensure their safety and efficacy before they can be widely adopted in clinical settings.

3D bioprinting holds a significant promise for cartilage repair in joints by creating scaffolds that closely mimic the native cartilage structure. This technology could revolutionize the treatment of joint disorders and injuries. However, ongoing research, addressing challenges in mechanical properties and integration, and navigating regulatory landscapes are essential for translating this technology into clinical practice.

Organ Transplantation: Kidneys, Liver, and Heart

Kidneys and Bioprinting

The kidney is a highly complex organ, responsible for vital functions such as filtering blood, removing waste, balancing electrolytes, and regulating blood pressure. Its intricate structure includes numerous cell types, such as nephrons (the functional units), blood vessels, and supporting tissues. Replicating this complexity is one of the significant challenges in bioprinting kidneys.

Despite these challenges, there have been notable advancements in bioprinting renal tissues. Researchers have been focusing on creating smaller segments of the kidney, such as nephrons, to understand and replicate the organ's functionality.

The ultimate goal of bioprinting kidneys is to produce fully functional organs for transplantation. This would address the critical shortage of donor kidneys. While a fully bioprinted, transplantable kidney has not yet been achieved, progress in this area could revolutionize treatment for kidney failure.

Bioprinted renal tissues are also valuable for disease modeling and drug testing. They can be used to study kidney diseases at a cellular level, test new drugs, and understand the progression of renal conditions.[24]

This application is particularly crucial, given the complexity of kidney diseases and the limitations of current models.

A notable example is the work by researchers at the Wake Forest Institute for Regenerative Medicine, who have made progress in bioprinting human kidney cells and structures that mimic the natural organ.[25]

Another example is the development of mini-kidneys or kidney organoids.

A kidney organoid is a 3D cluster of cells, cultivated from stem cells in a laboratory setting, that naturally arranges itself in a way that mimics normal kidney development. This process results in the formation of nephron structures, which closely resemble those found in a natural kidney organ.[26]

These organoids offer a model for studying kidney development and disease.

One of the major challenges in kidney bioprinting is ensuring adequate vascularization — the formation of blood vessels — within the printed tissue. This is crucial for the survival and functionality of the bioprinted kidney.

Replicating the full functionality of the kidney, including its ability to filter blood and produce urine, remains a significant hurdle.

As with all organ bioprinting endeavors, there are regulatory and ethical considerations to navigate, especially concerning clinical trials and transplantation protocols.

Liver

The liver is known for its remarkable regenerative capabilities, making it a prime candidate for bioprinting applications. Unlike many other organs, the liver can regenerate itself even after significant portions have been damaged or removed. This unique characteristic provides a solid foundation for developing bioprinted liver tissues.

The primary goal of liver bioprinting is to create functional liver tissue for transplantation. This is particularly crucial given the high demand for liver transplants and the shortage of donor organs. Bioprinted liver tissues could potentially alleviate this shortage and provide a lifesaving solution for patients with liver failure.

Drug Testing

Bioprinted liver tissues can be used to test the toxicity and efficacy of new drugs.[27]

The liver plays a critical role in metabolizing medications, and bio-printed tissues can provide a more accurate representation of how drugs will behave in the human body compared to traditional cell cultures or animal models.[28]

Organovo has developed bioprinted liver tissues that are used for drug toxicity testing, providing a more accurate model of human liver responses.[29]

Disease Study

These tissues can also be used to model liver diseases, such as hepatitis or cirrhosis, allowing for a better understanding of these conditions and the development of new treatments.

Organovo, a biotechnology company, has also been at the forefront of developing bioprinted liver tissues for disease modeling. They have successfully created liver tissues that can survive and function for extended periods in vitro.

The liver's complex vascular structure and diverse cell types pose significant challenges in bioprinting. Achieving the precise arrangement of cells and vascular networks is essential for creating functional liver tissue.[26]

Ensuring the long-term functionality and integration of bioprinted liver tissues within the human body also remains a major hurdle.

Heart

Bioprinting heart tissue involves creating cardiac patches that can be applied to damaged heart tissue, offering potential treatments for heart disease and failure.

Example: Researchers at the Tel Aviv University successfully printed a small-scale heart using human cells, a significant step toward full heart bioprinting.[30]

Bioprinting in the context of heart tissue primarily focuses on creating cardiac patches. These patches are engineered pieces of tissue designed to be applied to damaged areas of the heart. They are intended to integrate with the existing cardiac tissue, supporting or restoring its function. This approach is particularly promising for treating heart disease and heart failure, where damaged heart tissue often cannot regenerate on its own.[31]

These bioprinted cardiac patches typically contain a combination of cardiac cells, including cardiomyocytes (heart muscle cells), endothelial cells (which line blood vessels), and smooth muscle cells. The aim is to mimic the natural structure and function of heart tissue, including its unique electrical conductivity and contractility.

Applications in Treatment and Research

For patients with heart disease or those who have suffered a heart attack, bioprinted cardiac patches could provide a novel treatment option by repairing the damaged heart tissue and improving heart function.

Like liver and kidney bioprinting, bioprinted heart tissues can be used for drug testing and modeling heart diseases. This allows for a better understanding of cardiac conditions and the development of targeted therapies.[32]

A study by Ong et al.[33] in the *Journal of Thoracic Disease* discussed the potential of 3D bioprinting for cardiac repair by delivering stem cells to the damaged heart tissue using 3D bioprinted cardiac patches.

Challenges and Future Directions

One of the main challenges is replicating the complex functionality of heart tissue, including its electrical conductivity and ability to contract in a synchronized manner.

Ensuring adequate vascularization within the bioprinted tissue and its successful integration with the patient's existing heart tissue are critical for the functionality of the cardiac patches.

Navigating the regulatory landscape for clinical application and addressing ethical concerns are essential for the advancement of bio-printed heart tissues into clinical practice.

Bioprinting heart tissue, particularly in the form of cardiac patches, offers potential treatments for heart disease and failure. While significant challenges remain in replicating the full functionality of heart tissue and ensuring successful integration, the advancements in this field are promising and could lead to groundbreaking treatments for cardiac conditions.

Personalized Medicine: Patient-Specific Implants and Grafts

3D bioprinting is revolutionizing personalized medicine by enabling the creation of patient-specific implants and grafts.[34]

This approach ensures a higher compatibility and reduces the risk of rejection and complications.

1. Customized Implants: Using patient-specific data from imaging techniques such as MRI or CT scans, implants can be tailored to fit the unique anatomy of each patient. This is particularly useful in reconstructive surgery and orthopedics.
2. Tissue Grafts: Bioprinted tissue grafts, customized to match the patient's tissues, can be used in various reconstructive procedures, offering improved outcomes compared to traditional grafts.

In summary, 3D organ printing holds immense potential across various medical fields, from creating complex tissues for repair and regeneration to developing patient-specific implants and advancing organ transplantation. As the technology continues to evolve, its impact on medicine is expected to grow, offering new solutions to previously insurmountable challenges.

Current State of the Art in Bioprinting

In terms of notable achievements, the field has seen significant strides in creating complex tissue structures, including the development of vascular networks and multilayered skin, crucial for larger organ functionality. By printing vascular cells and appropriate biomaterial scaffolding, 3D printing can mimic in vivo conditions to generate blood vessels.[35]

The creation of organoids and mini-organs has also been a break-through, offering new avenues for disease modeling, drug testing, and understanding organ development.[36]

Additionally, the bioprinting of functional tissue patches, especially for cardiac and liver tissues, stands out as a promising area for organ repair.

Successful applications of 3D bioprinting are diverse. Skin bioprint-ing, for instance, has shown immense potential in regenerating skin for burn victims, allowing for the customization of grafts to match specific wound characteristics. 3D bioprinting for treating burn injuries uses a process where cells and scaffolding materials are meticulously deposited layer by layer onto the injured area. This technique can be performed in two different ways: in situ or in vitro. The primary difference between these approaches lies in the location of the printing and the subsequent maturation of the tissue. In situ, bioprinting involves directly applying the bioink layers onto the wound site, allowing the tissue to develop and inte-grate in its natural location. In contrast, in vitro, bioprinting is carried out in a controlled laboratory environment, where the skin tissue is developed externally before being transplanted to the injury site. Despite this differ-ence in location, both methods follow a similar fundamental process of layering cells and scaffold materials to reconstruct the damaged skin.

In orthopedics, bioprinted cartilage scaffolds have been explored for joint repair, particularly beneficial for osteoarthritis patients or those with traumatic injuries. Dental applications of bioprinting, including the crea-tion of dental implants and complex structures such as periodontal tissue, have also been a focus of recent research.

However, the field faces several limitations and challenges. Vascularization remains a significant hurdle in bioprinting larger tissues and organs, as creating an adequate blood supply is crucial for tissue sur-vival and function. Ensuring cell viability and functionality over the long term within bioprinted structures is another major challenge. Material limitations also pose a problem, as finding materials that balance mechan-ical stability with biocompatibility is complex. These materials must sup-port essential cellular processes such as attachment, proliferation, and differentiation. Ethical and regulatory issues concerning the use of human cells and the clinical application of bioprinted tissues and organs are ongoing. Additionally, the high cost and technical expertise required for bioprinting technologies limit their widespread use and accessibility.

Ethical and Regulatory Considerations

In the realm of 3D bioprinting, ethical and regulatory considerations play a pivotal role, especially given the technology's potential to revolutionize medical treatments and organ transplantation. These considerations are crucial in ensuring that the development and application of bioprinted tissues and organs are conducted responsibly and safely.

The ethical implications of bioprinting human tissues and organs are multifaceted. One primary concern is the source of cells used in bioprinting.[37]

The use of stem cells, particularly embryonic stem cells, raises ethical questions regarding the origin and consent for use. Additionally, there are concerns about the long-term effects and potential unintended consequences of implanting bioprinted tissues and organs in humans. Issues such as the potential for organ rejection, unforeseen biological responses, and the long-term viability of the bioprinted organs need careful ethical consideration. Furthermore, there is a debate over access and equity in the distribution of these potentially lifesaving technologies, ensuring that advancements in bioprinting do not exacerbate existing healthcare inequalities.

The regulatory landscape for 3D printed organs and tissues is still evolving. Regulatory bodies such as the U.S. Food and Drug Administration (FDA) are tasked with ensuring that bioprinted products are safe and effective for clinical use. This involves rigorous testing and validation processes. The FDA has been developing guidelines and standards for 3D bioprinting, but the novelty and complexity of the technology pose unique challenges.[38]

These include determining the appropriate regulatory pathways, standards for manufacturing and quality control, and guidelines for clinical trials. The regulatory framework must be flexible enough to accommodate rapid technological advancements while ensuring patient safety and efficacy.

Patient safety is paramount in the application of bioprinted tissues and organs.[39]

This involves ensuring that bioprinted products are free from contamination, structurally sound, and functionally effective. Quality control measures must be stringent, from the selection and handling of cells to the final implantation of bioprinted tissues or organs. This includes rigorous testing for biocompatibility, durability, and functionality. Additionally, long-term monitoring and follow-up are essential to assess the success of bioprinted implants and to gather data for continuous improvement of the technology.

While 3D bioprinting holds immense potential in the field of regenerative medicine, navigating the ethical and regulatory landscape is crucial for its responsible development and application. Ensuring patient safety through stringent quality control measures is a fundamental aspect of this journey. As technology advances, continuous dialogue among scientists, ethicists, regulators, and the public will be essential to address these complex issues effectively.

Conclusion

The impact of 3D organ printing in the field of medicine and healthcare is both profound and far-reaching. This innovative technology, at the intersection of engineering, biology, and medicine, holds the promise of revolutionizing organ transplantation and tissue repair. It offers hope for addressing the chronic shortage of donor organs and provides new avenues for personalized medicine, where treatments and medical solutions are tailored to the individual needs of patients.

The ability to print complex tissues and organs layer by layer, with precision and customization, opens possibilities for treating a wide range of medical conditions, from burn injuries and bone defects to heart disease and liver failure. The advancements in this field have already shown significant potential, particularly in creating skin grafts, cartilage for joint repair, and functional tissue patches for damaged organs.

However, the journey ahead is not without its challenges. The complexity of replicating the intricate structures and functions of human organs, ensuring long-term viability and integration of bioprinted tissues, and overcoming hurdles in vascularization remains significant scientific challenges. Additionally, the ethical and regulatory landscape surrounding the use of bioprinted organs and tissues is complex and evolving. Ensuring patient safety, equitable access to these advanced treatments, and navigating the ethical implications of using human cells for printing tissues and organs are critical considerations that must be addressed as the technology progresses.

Despite these challenges, the opportunities presented by 3D organ printing are immense. As research and development in this field continue to advance, we can anticipate more breakthroughs that will push the boundaries of what is currently possible in medical science. The potential for improving patient outcomes, reducing the burden on organ donation systems, and enhancing the efficacy of medical treatments is substantial.

In summary, 3D organ printing stands at the forefront of a new era in healthcare, offering exciting prospects for the future. The path forward will require a collaborative effort among scientists, medical professionals, ethicists, and policymakers to fully realize the potential of this groundbreaking technology while addressing the challenges and ethical considerations that come with it.

References

1. Albanna M, Binder KW, Murphy SV, Kim J, Qasem SA, Zhao W, et al. In situ bioprinting of autologous skin cells accelerates wound healing of extensive excisional full-thickness wounds. *Sci Rep.* 2019;9(1):1856. doi:10.1038/s41598-018-38366-w.
2. Rajabi N, Rezaei A, Kharaziha M, Bakhsheshi-Rad HR, Luo H, RamaKrishna S, Berto F. Recent advances on bioprinted gelatin methacrylate-based hydrogels for tissue repair. *Tissue Eng Part A.* 2021;27(11–12):679–702. doi:10.1089/ten.TEA.2020.0350.
3. Gao G, Schilling AF, Yonezawa T, Wang J, Dai G, Cui X. Bioactive nanoparticles stimulate bone tissue formation in bioprinted three-dimensional scaffold and human mesenchymal stem cells. *Biotechnol J.* 2014 Oct;9(10):1304–1311. doi:10.1002/biot.201400305. Epub 2014 Sep 10. PMID: 25130390.

4. Skylar-Scott MA, Uzel SGM, Nam LL, Ahrens JH, Truby RL, Damaraju S, et al. Biomanufacturing of organ-specific tissues with high cellular density and embedded vascular channels. *Sci Adv*. 2019 Sep 6;5(9):eaaw2459. doi:10.1126/sciadv.aaw2459. PMID: 31523707; PMCID: PMC6731072.

5. Kang HW, Lee SJ, Ko IK, Kengla C, Yoo JJ, Atala A. A 3D bioprinting system to produce human-scale tissue constructs with structural integrity. *Nat Biotechnol*. 2016;34(3):312–319. doi:10.1038/nbt.3413.

6. Murphy SV, Atala A. 3D bioprinting of tissues and organs. *Nat Biotechnol*. 2014;32(8):773–785. doi:10.1038/nbt.2958.

7. Jessop ZM, Al-Sabah A, Gardiner MD, Combellack E, Hawkins K, Whitaker IS. 3D bioprinting for reconstructive surgery: principles, applications and challenges. *J Plast, Reconstr Aesthet Surg*. 2017;70(9):1155–1170. doi:10.1016/j.bjps.2017.06.006.

8. Cohen DL, Lipton JI, Bonassar LJ, Lipson H. Additive manufacturing for in situ repair of osteochondral defects. *Biofabrication*. 2010;2(3):035004. doi:10.1088/1758-5082/2/3/035004.

9. Guillotin B, Souquet A, Catros S, Pippenger B, Bellance S, Bareille R, et al. Laser-assisted bioprinting of engineered tissue with high cell density and microscale organization. *Biomaterials*. 2010;31(28):7250–7256. doi:10.1016/j.biomaterials.2010.05.055.

10. Hospodiuk M, Dey M, Sosnoski D, Ozbolat IT. The bioink: a comprehensive review on bioprintable materials. *Biotechnol Adv*. 2017;35(2):217–239. doi:10.1016/j.biotechadv.2016.12.006.

11. Zhang YS, Arneri A, Bersini S, Shin SR, Zhu K, Goli-Malekabadi Z, et al. Bioprinting 3D microfibrous scaffolds for engineering endothelialized myocardium and heart-on-a-chip. *Biomaterials*. 2016;110:45–59. doi:10.1016/j.biomaterials.2016.09.003.

12. Cubo N, Garcia M, Del Cañizo JF, Velasco D, Jorcano JL. 3D bioprinting of functional human skin: production and in vivo analysis. *Biofabrication*. 2016 Dec 5;9(1):015006. doi:10.1088/1758-5090/9/1/015006. PMID: 27917823.

13. Cooper GM, Miller ED, Decesare GE, Usas A, Lensie EL, Bykowski MR, et al. Inkjet-based biopatterning of bone morphogenetic protein-2 to spatially control calvarial bone formation. *Tissue Eng Part A*. 2010 May;16(5):1749–1759. doi:10.1089/ten.TEA.2009.0650. PMID: 20028232; PMCID: PMC2952127.

14. Do AV, Khorsand B, Geary SM, Salem AK. 3D printing of scaffolds for tissue regeneration applications. *Adv Healthc Mater*. 2015 Aug 26;4(12):1742–1762. doi:10.1002/adhm.201500168. Epub 2015 Jun 10. PMID: 26097108; PMCID: PMC4597933.

15. Lee S, Matsugaki A, Kasuga T, Nakano T. Development of bifunctional oriented bioactive glass/poly(lactic acid) composite scaffolds to control osteoblast alignment and proliferation. *J Biomed Mater Res Part A.* 2019;107A:1031–1041.

16. Ginebra MP, Espanol M, Maazouz Y, Bergez V, Pastorino D. Bioceramics and bone healing. *EFORT Open Rev.* 2018 May 21;3(5):173–183. doi:10.1302/2058-5241.3.170056. PMID: 29951254; PMCID: PMC5994622.

17. Urist MR, Lietze A, Dawson E. Beta-tricalcium phosphate delivery system for bone morphogenetic protein. *Clin Orthop Relat Res.* 1984;187:277–280.

18. Valentini P, Abensur D, Wenz B, Peetz M, Schenk R. Sinus grafting with porous bone mineral (Bio-Oss) for implant placement: a 5-year study on 15 patients. *Int J Periodontics Restorative Dent.* 2000;20(3):245–253.

19. Xue J, Qin C, Wu C. 3D printing of cell-delivery scaffolds for tissue regeneration. *Regen Biomater.* 2023 Mar 27;10:rbad032. doi:10.1093/rb/rbad032. PMID: 37081861; PMCID: PMC10112960.

20. Daly AC, Cunniffe GM, Sathy BN, Jeon O, Alsberg E, Kelly DJ. 3D bioprinting of developmentally inspired templates for whole bone organ engineering. *Adv Healthc Mater.* 2017;6(17):1700935. https://doi.org/10.1002/adhm.201600182.

21. Daly AC, Kelly DJ. Biofabrication of spatially organized tissues by directing the growth of cellular spheroids within 3D printed polymeric microchambers. *Biomaterials.* 2019;197:194–206. doi:10.1016/j.biomaterials.2018.12.028.

22. Mouser VHM, Levato R, Bonassar LJ, D'Lima DD, Grande DA, Klein TJ, et al. Three-dimensional bioprinting and its potential in the field of articular cartilage regeneration. *Cartilage.* 2017;8(4):327–340. doi:10.1177/1947603516665445.

23. Xu Y, Chen C, Hellwarth PB, Bao X. Biomaterials for stem cell engineering and biomanufacturing. *Bioact Mater.* 2019 Dec 2;4:366–379.

24. Fransen MFJ, Addario G, Bouten CVC, Halary F, Moroni L, Mota C. Bioprinting of kidney in vitro models: cells, biomaterials, and manufacturing techniques. *Essays Biochem.* 2021 Aug 10;65(3):587–602. doi:10.1042/EBC20200158. PMID: 34096573; PMCID: PMC8365327.

25. Wake Forest University. *Engineering a Kidney.* https://school.wakehealth.edu/research/institutes-and-centers/wake-forest-institute-for-regenerative-medicine/research/replacement-organs-and-tissue/engineering-a-kidney. Accessed 2024 Jan 26.

26. Chambers BE, Weaver NE, Wingert RA. The "3Ds" of growing kidney organoids: advances in nephron development, disease modeling, and drug screening. *Cells*. 2023 Feb 8;12(4):549. doi:10.3390/cells12040549. PMID: 36831216; PMCID: PMC9954122.

27. Li W, Liu Z, Tang F, Jiang H, Zhou Z, Hao X, et al. Application of 3D bioprinting in liver diseases. *Micromachines (Basel)*. 2023 Aug 21;14(8):1648. doi:10.3390/mi14081648. PMID: 37630184; PMCID: PMC10457767.

28. Kamimura H, Ito S. Assessment of chimeric mice with humanized livers in new drug development: generation of pharmacokinetics, metabolism and toxicity data for selecting the final candidate compound. *Xenobiotica*. 2016;46:557–569. doi:10.3109/00498254.2015.1091113.

29. Organovo. ExVive™ 3D bioprinted human liver tissue for modeling progressive liver disease. Organovo Website. 2017. https://organovo.com/3d-bioprinted-human-liver-tissue-modeling-progressive-liver-disease/. Accessed 2024 Jan 24.

30. Noor N, Shapira A, Edri R, Gal I, Wertheim L, Dvir T. 3D printing of personalized thick and perfusable cardiac patches and hearts. *Adv Sci (Weinh)*. 2019 Apr 15;6(11):1900344. doi:10.1002/advs.201900344. PMID: 31179230; PMCID: PMC6548966.

31. Rosellini E, Cascone MG, Guidi L, Schubert DW, Roether JA, Boccaccini AR. Mending a broken heart by biomimetic 3D printed natural biomaterial-based cardiac patches: a review. *Front Bioeng Biotechnol*. 2023 Nov 16;11:1254739. doi:10.3389/fbioe.2023.1254739. PMID: 38047285; PMCID: PMC10690428.

32. Gardin C, Ferroni L, Latremouille C, Chachques JC, Mitrečić D, Zavan B. Recent applications of three-dimensional printing in cardiovascular medicine. *Cells*. 2020 Mar 17;9(3):742. doi:10.3390/cells9030742. PMID: 32192232; PMCID: PMC7140676.

33. Ong CS, Fukunishi T, Zhang H, Huang CY, Nashed A, Blazeski A, et al. Biomaterial-free three-dimensional bioprinting of cardiac tissue using human induced pluripotent stem cell-derived cardiomyocytes. *Sci Rep*. 2017;7(1):4566. doi:10.1038/s41598-017-05018-4.

34. Shopova D, Yaneva A, Bakova D, Mihaylova A, Kasnakova P, Hristozova M, et al. (Bio)printing in personalized medicine-opportunities and potential benefits. *Bioengineering (Basel)*. 2023 Feb 23;10(3):287. doi:10.3390/bioengineering10030287. PMID: 36978678; PMCID: PMC10045778.

35. Jafarkhani M, Salehi Z, Aidun A, Shokrgozar MA. Bioprinting in vascularization strategies. *Iran Biomed J*. 2019 Jan;23(1):9–20. doi:10.29252/.23.1.9. PMID: 30458600; PMCID: PMC6305822.

36. Lee H. Engineering In vitro models: bioprinting of organoids with artificial intelligence. *Cyborg Bionic Syst.* 2023;4:0018. doi:10.34133/cbsystems.0018. Epub 2023 Mar 29. PMID: 37011281; PMCID: PMC10057937.

37. Kirillova A, Bushev S, Abubakirov A, Sukikh G. Bioethical and legal Issues in 3D bioprinting. *Int J Bioprint.* 2020 Apr 28;6(3):272. doi:10.18063/ijb.v6i3.272. PMID: 33088986; PMCID: PMC7557521.

38. Pew. *FDA's Regulatory Framework for 3D Printing of Medical Devices at the Point of Care Needs More Clarity.* 2022. https://www.pewtrusts.org/en/research-and-analysis/issue-briefs/2022/07/fdas-regulatory-framework-for-3d-printing-of-medical-devices-needs-more-clarity. Accessed 2024 Jan 26.

39. Ricci G, Gibelli F, Sirignano A. Three-dimensional bioprinting of human organs and tissues: bioethical and medico-legal implications examined through a scoping review. *Bioengineering (Basel).* 2023 Sep 7;10(9):1052. doi:10.3390/bioengineering10091052. PMID: 37760154; PMCID: PMC10525297.

Conclusion

Realizing the Full Potential of Medical Technology

As we have explored in this book, the landscape of medical technology is rapidly evolving, offering unprecedented opportunities to enhance patient care. From the expansion of telemedicine to the cutting-edge developments in genomics and precision medicine, these advancements promise to revolutionize healthcare. However, realizing the full potential of these technologies requires a balanced approach that synthesizes their benefits while managing inherent risks and challenges.

Integrating telemedicine and virtual care has shown us the possibilities of remote patient monitoring and care beyond traditional hospital settings. This shift improves access and convenience and plays a crucial role in reducing contagion risks, as seen in recent global health crises. Yet, it is essential to maintain personal connections between patients and healthcare providers, overcoming the limitations of virtual interactions.

Artificial intelligence (AI) and big data are transforming the diagnosis and treatment landscape. Using AI for precision diagnosis, treatment recommendations, and predictions is a significant leap forward. However, ensuring the accuracy of these tools, removing biases, and maintaining human oversight are critical to avoid misdiagnoses and ensure ethical use. Protecting patient data privacy and security in this era of big data is also paramount.

The advent of robotics and procedural automation, particularly in surgeries and routine tasks, is another area of rapid advancement. While robots assist in surgeries and automate tasks, it is vital to maintain physician training and oversight to ensure the quality of care. The development of robotics for rehabilitation and prosthetics is a promising field that could significantly impact patient recovery and quality of life.

In genomics and precision medicine, the sequencing of individual genomes and the use of pharmacogenetics are paving the way for highly personalized care. Employing biomarkers to customize treatments and predict outcomes is an exciting development, but making genomics affordable and accessible remains challenging. Additionally, safeguarding privacy in collecting and using genetic data is a critical concern.

The emergence of organs-on-a-chip, wearable monitors, and mHealth applications represents the next frontier in medical technology. These innovations can potentially personalize healthcare further and provide real-time health monitoring, offering new disease prevention and management insights.

Collaborative oversight and physician responsibility are crucial to synthesizing the benefits of these technological advancements. As we embrace these innovations, prioritizing personalized care, empathy, and the human element in medicine is essential. The goal should be building a more ethical, transparent, patient-centered healthcare system.

The future of medical technology is bright and holds immense promise for improving patient outcomes and healthcare delivery. However, this future must be navigated with a keen awareness of medicine's ethical, practical, and human aspects. By maintaining a focus on personalized care and empathy, ensuring rigorous oversight and continuous physician education, and addressing challenges such as accessibility, privacy, and equity, we can harness the full potential of medical technology. This approach will advance healthcare and ensure that it remains compassionate, patient-centered, and true to medicine's core values.

Index

abacavir, 153, 166

Accreditation Commission for Health Care (ACHC), 64

additive manufacturing, 208

Adler, 90

advanced visualization, 92

adverse drug reactions, 147, 153, 166

AI algorithms, 2

AI and machine learning (ML), 154

AI-assisted surgical planning, 23

Alone Together: Why We Expect More from Technology and Less from Each Other, 113

AlphaGo, 94

American Civil War, 46

American College of Medical Genetics and Genomics, 152

American Telemedicine Association (ATA), 48, 64

Apple's iPhone, 48

Apple Watch, 129

assistive robots, 100

AsthmaMD, 135

augmented decision-making, 29

augmenting healthcare professionals, 5

authentication and access controls, 69

automation of routine tasks, 28

autonomous, 89

Balkan conflicts, 48

best practices, 57

bioactive glass foam, 218

bioceramics, 224

biocompatibility, 211, 216

biodegradability, 216

biodegradable polymer foam, 218

bioinks, 210
    compatibility with, 215
    creating, 220

biomaterial developments, 196

biomedical telemetry, 47

bioprinters, 213

bioprinting, 208
    extrusion-based, 214
    inkjet-based, 213
    laser-assisted, 215

bone, 223
    bioprinting, 223
    bone morphogenetic proteins (BMPs), 223

brain-on-a-chip, 190, 195